SAME TIME
NEXT WEEK?

She Lives!
The Berkowitz Diet Switch
(with Gerald Berkowitz, M.D.)
The Virile Man
(with Sheldon Fellman, M.D.)
Wilderness World
(four volumes)
The Key to Better Health
A Sensible Approach to Dieting
(with Eugene Scheimann, M.D.)
A Doctor Discusses Back Problems
(with Gerald Berkowitz, M.D.)
Female Surgery
(with Samuel Matlin, M.D.)
Goodbye, Loneliness
(with J. H. Schmidt, M.D.)
All About You
Minimizing Post-Partum Problems
(with Bernice Rosen, M.D.)
The Best Time
Blackthink
(with Jesse Owens)
I Have Changed
(with Jesse Owens)
The Jesse Owens Story
(with Jesse Owens)
Jesse: The Man Who Outran Hitler
(with Jesse Owens)
How to Be Lucky
(with Philip John Neimark)
John Wayne's Secret
A Medical Approach to Alcoholism
Four Weekends to An Ideal Marriage
(with Herbert Glieberman)
Closed Marriage
(with Herbert Glieberman)
Sex and the Overnight Woman
(with Eugene Scheimann, M.D.)
Staying Youthful
Getting Along
(with J. H. Schmidt, M.D.)

Same Time Next Week?

by PAUL NEIMARK

with an introduction by
Stanford R. Gamm, M. D.

ARLINGTON HOUSE PUBLISHERS
Westport, Connecticut

Special thanks to
a Special man—
Marc Konsler

Because of the inviolable confidentiality of the
psychotherapeutic-patient relationship, each conversation
and comment quoted in SAME TIME NEXT WEEK?,
unless specifically attributed to specific individuals, is a
representative mixture of several or many conversations
and comments, and not attributable to any specific
individual.

Library of Congress Cataloging in Publication Data

Neimark, Paul G.
    Same time next week

    1. Psychotherapist and patient.   2. Psychotherapy—
Decision making.   3. Patient education.   I. Title.
RC480.8.N44   616.89'14   81-10818
ISBN 0-87000-514-6   AACR2
Production Services by Cobb/Dunlop, Inc.
9 8 7 6 5 4 3 2

TO PHIL,
his own therapist

Contents

CONTENTS

Foreword

Today psychotherapy is practiced by psychiatric physicians, psychologists, social workers, pastoral counselors, and others with various theoretical orientations, techniques, and goals.

The outcome of psychotherapy depends upon many factors, including those of the patient, the therapist, and the relationship between them. The nature and severity of the patient's problem must be considered significant. The training, experience, skill, and personality of the therapist have much weight. In the final analysis, it is the nature and workability of the patient-therapist relationship that determines the result.

For me, successful psychotherapy depends on a delicate, unique, and highly personal patient-therapist relationship. Therapy will usually affect the therapist as well as the patient. Both will grow in the relationship, the patient more than the therapist, because hopefully the therapist is already more resolved and mature. A good therapeutic relationship needs much empathy, introspection, and positive regard. The therapist provides an atmosphere of confidentiality, openness, and trust, which encourages the patient to confide her or his thoughts and feelings more openly over time. The therapist generally does not reveal her or his own thoughts and feelings to the patient freely unless in her or his best judgment it would be helpful to the patient to do so. Thus, it might be prudent for the therapist to show the patient that the therapist is human, makes mistakes sometimes, and occasionally has troubled feelings too, provided it does not burden the patient. Such decisions require intuitive and trained knowledge on the part of the therapist.

In the course of time the patient develops more or less dependence on the therapist and their sessions together. The therapist becomes attuned to this and handles it in the patient's best interest. With both patient and therapist open to each other and the therapeutic process (as the ideal), therapy may occur daily, several times a week, weekly, biweekly, monthly, and in varying combinations, depending on the patient's needs. Therapy may require only a few sessions over a short period of time (the exception), or may last months, years, or indefinitely.

Psychotherapy can be a very difficult, slow process. There may be relapses and stalemates. Some patients change markedly, some less. Some do better with one therapist, some with another. Therapeutic fit is important. Some patients do well with one therapist for a while, then need to change to another. Some do better with one therapist throughout their therapy. Therapy is not easy for either patient or therapist. In fact, it may be hard work and at times quite painful. But usually it is very much worth the effort. Therapy depends less on theories and diagnostic labels than on the capacity of the therapist to be skillfully observant, empathic, and introspective. And it helps when they can provide a corrective relationship of a positive presence. Since we deal with problems that have no definitive answers, there are no "cures." But there are definite improvements, sometimes lifesaving and life-enhancing, of profound dimensions.

There are no supertherapists, just psychiatrically educated human beings who might help people but at least don't harm them. Therapists' ego problems, especially their omnipotence and narcissism, are the main culprits in interfering with a patient's progress.

Psychotherapy is both an art and a science. It is a science to the extent that it is based on time-tested hypotheses of the biological, psychological, and social sciences. It is an art to the extent that it attempts to deal creatively with unique subjective human emotions, values, and experiences we all share to some extent, but which cannot as yet be quantified, predicted, or duplicated.

Philosophically, psychotherapy is a humanistic, democratic endeavor, an open dialogue between individuals who work together without coercion for a common goal, to help a fellow human being become a better person, effective but not arrogant, independent but not aloof, tolerant but with high ideals, understanding without being permissive or seductive, and appropriately loving.

The one thing I know about the author that would qualify him to write a book on psychotherapy is that he asks very pertinent and penetrating questions about it. That does not mean that he has the answers—nor do I necessarily. Nor does anyone.

STANFORD R. GAMM, M.D.

A lot of people, especially this one psychoanalyst guy they have here, keeps asking me if I'm going to apply myself when I go back to school next September. It's such a stupid question, in my opinion. I mean how do you know what you're going to do till you do it? The answer is, you don't. I think I am, but how do I know? I swear it's a stupid question.

J. D. SALINGER

Catcher In The Rye

SAME TIME
NEXT WEEK?

1
Why This Book Came to Be

This book was born because I had to know what Anne knew.

Thoreau, at the outset of *Walden,* explained that he was writing in the first person, not for the usual reasons, but because he himself was the person with whom he was most familiar. By the same token, I devote this chapter to my wife and myself, not because I want to, but because I should.

A book on this subject must, above all, in fairness to the reader, identify the author psychologically as well as biographically.

What does qualify me if I am not a therapist? Have I been in therapy myself? How did I come to write a book such as this? What are my sources? What are my standards of evaluation? The answers to these and related questions are inextricably part of the book itself.

First, I am qualified because I am *not* "qualified."

Today you and I find ourselves in a mind-bogglingly complex, specialized world. If we need our taxes done, we go to an accountant, if we wish to invest in stocks, we go to a broker—seldom questioning whether he *really* knows better. And we almost always give a blank check to the specialist. This is especially true when there is "Dr." before someone's name, because doctor is the "specialty" that deals with the bottom line of our existence: our physical and mental health. Partly because doctors do deal with that which is most fundamental to us (and partly because America's awe for long years of formal education and the degrees that accompany them), Dr. before a man or woman's name has acquired a transcendent authority.

Nothing might be known about a doctor's sexual life, for example—he may be a dud in bed or someone with extreme sexual problems—but if he puts his name to a book with a clever format, appealing style or big promotion campaign, he'll become a leading "expert" on sex.

Or on dieting, even though he's never really had a problem with overweight himself, or doesn't know much more about the subject than most of the rest of us.

Or on relieving tension, even though he's never been able to relieve his own.

What does "Dr." *really* mean, particulary in reference to psychotherapy? Could it mean opportunist? Safe-player? Genius? Witch doctor? *That* is one of the things this book is about, and is the prime reason why such a book cannot and should not be written by a ... doctor.

A second reason this book should be written by an "outsider" is that it would be next to impossible for a doctor to write it. A physician, who has no more claim to psychiatric expertise than anyone else, by nature and because of powerful medical and state laws, plus the mushrooming threat of malpractice suits, is seldom a boat-rocker. The therapist has an added confinement: His relationships are confidential, his information privileged. A handful of therapists, it is true, *have* written for their patients rather than for their colleagues, and a few, notably Dr. Richard Chessick in his wise and courageous *Why Psychotherapists Fail,* have been openly critical of their profession. Still, they cannot, on the bottom line, pivot from the patient's viewpoint.

Though I was born into a "family of doctors," I never wanted to be one. My grandfather was a leading allergist, my father is a fine dentist who later narrated a daily TV dental clinic for the public, plus various cousins and uncles in the medical profession. My father would have become a doctor if his family had had enough money. Actually, he might have become a baseball player—he was offered a contract with the Chicago White Sox—but his mother insisted he go into a profession. My grandfather really practiced psychology more than medicine, prescribing placebos more often than pills. He knew that doctoring the mind was the new frontier, and our home was usually filled with physicians and psychiatrists. From my earliest recollection I had the opportunity to listen and talk to them. Dr. Walter Alvarez, former Chief Consultant at the Mayo Clinic and author of numerous books on psychosomatic medicine, was one. Jules Masserman and Lionel Blitzen were familiar friends of the family. I could not know what they were like as therapists—who can except the patient?—but I was able to observe them as human beings throughout the years.

Blitzen was a tiny, round, brilliant man with thick glasses that made his constant stare seem even more piercing. On the other hand, Masserman, whose name appears in the index of nearly every current book on psychotherapy, was friendly and jovial. My mother feels he is a great man, and he may be.

I also had the chance to observe firsthand subsequent events in the lives of many of the patients of other therapists I met. By the time I left my parents' home at twenty for marriage and my own home, I had formed two conclusions. First, most therapists couldn't seem to solve their own personal problems, so I wondered how they could solve those of their patients. Second, most patients whom I observed or knew of were not only no better from therapy, but seemingly, worse for it. I worshiped the ideal of the medical profession and those who attempted to attain it. But I had come to agree with my grandfather's appraisal that most therapists couldn't help themselves, let alone others, and that, in general, doctors "kill nine for every one we cure."

Anne began therapy when she was twenty-nine. We had been married ten years, and she had developed agoraphobia (which, as far as I am concerned, may well be a rational reaction to the world), stemming from a bitter divorce by her parents when she was nine. She was not allowed to see her father and lived alone with her mother, to whom she had frequently and crucially to be more the mother than the daughter.

Anne is a remarkable argument against virtually everything in this book asserted against psychotherapy and psychotherapists. She loves therapy; it has helped her. One reason for this is that she remarkably combines rationality and grit. Even though she was in extreme suffering when she began looking for a good therapist, Anne didn't settle for anyone *less* than *good.* In life, and especially in therapy, most of us want our pain allayed at almost any cost. Instead, Anne visited therapist after therapist one time each—from a kindly older man who obviously wasn't at all up to the task to a manipulative opportunist whose money-making modus operandi was to maim emotionally —until she settled on ... the wrong one.

She stayed with this therapist for over six years, though she definitively did not improve. A classic psychoanalyst, his basic feedback was "Why do you feel that?" Usually he said nothing. It's hard to make mistakes that way—except for the biggest mistake: not helping the patient. A brilliant but rather rigid fellow, he had come highly recommended by more than one person whom she knew well.

5

I had occasion to see them now and then and hear second-hand of their progress. I saw little, if any.

As each month and year passed, it became harder for Anne to leave this therapist. Finally, she had to face the fact that he was doing her no good, and that her treatment should be terminated. At the end of the last session he said only "Good-bye." For a time, though she was more anguished than ever over the agoraphobia, Anne saw no therapist. Better none than one who couldn't manage more than a "good-bye" after six years. She seriously considered the possibility that there might not be a therapist who was able to help her. Then, in 1971, she discovered Dr. Jules Gelperin.

A man of uncommon sense, Gelperin was a maverick who made his own rules. One was a fierce fidelity. Among other things, he had been happily married for thirty-five years. Another was autonomy. "No one has ever had a handle on me," he once observed. A third was a good cigar. I think that was the only thing that did have a handle on him.

Jules Gelperin combined the two qualities crucial for Anne: though they never saw each other socially outside the professional relationship, he was the strong and supportive father she had never really had, and he was also a pretty damn good therapist. He cut through the teleological and sociological cant to the core of what was really on his patient's mind, and often straight out gave what he thought was the answer, or the question. Sometimes he was wrong. But he believed enough in the autonomy of those facing him to feel they could decide for themselves. He once advised Anne, for example, to leave me because I was impossible to live with. He was right about my being impossible to live with; his mistake was that for Anne I am even more impossible to live without—and vice versa. Once Gelperin realized this, he advised her to stay with me. He was very much like the hero of James Dickey's *Deliverance*. Anne's dedication to her second book, *Sigmund Freud: The World Within,* appropriately reads: "To Jules Gelperin, M.D., who held the looking glass with skill and patience—and who kept it so finely polished."

In 1977, at sixty-two, Gelperin suffered a critical heart attack. He virtually leaped from intensive care back to his office. He refused to give up the cigars, of course, but everything else, from what he ate to the way he walked, had to be modified, and he was a man who could not be modified. Psychically and immunologically, I believe, something had finally gotten a handle on him. Less than two years later, after cancer took hold in his gut, he died. His wife died shortly after, for no apparent medical reason. The reason was that she could not live without Jules.

Though Anne would never have left Gelperin, it became increasingly apparent, in the final year or two, that he was going to leave her. Reluctantly, but assiduously, she began searching for another therapist. Recently, she finally found one.

Though Anne and I possess an identical sense of life, we

are often diametrically different in the way we approach life. Dr. Watson once began to read to Sherlock Holmes some sociological story in the newspaper. Holmes stopped him cold, saying that if something did not relate directly and intensely to his consuming concern of criminology, he had no time for it. By nature and by choice, I am with Holmes. I recognize that all knowlege is inextricably interrelated, but I only *care* about what is directly, intensely important to *me*. And because Anne is *most* important to me, everything about her therapy—and therapy in general—became directly and intensely important to me. Psychology, particularly the relationship of the mental to the physical, which is central to a majority of my nonfiction books and my one novel, had always been my consuming interest. But this was no longer enough. Now I had to know *everything* that Anne knew.

A teleplay of the sixties in which Sterling Hayden played the lead tells it best. Hayden is slotted for president in a futuristic society seemingly completely free and ideal, except that the subject of books is never discussed. They don't exist, though they did once; Hayden had seen them as a child, and he keeps rocking the boat over the objections of his only brother, who is afraid for him. The hero won't back down, and in the end is thrown into a cell where, when the clock reaches twelve, a ray gun through the bars will electrocute him. As the hours pass, even the thought of his own death is not as overwhelmingly depressing to Hayden as the fact that evil seems to have won. Then, with but seconds left, the door to his cell suddenly swings open and his brother is thrown inside!

"*Why?*" Hayden exclaims.

"Because . . . *I* had to know . . . what *you* knew," his brother answers. As the ray gun begins annihilating them both, Hayden turns to his executors and with complete conviction shouts, "You're going to lose . . . lose . . . *lose . . . .*"

I didn't want to lose. I wanted—want—to know and possess Anne totally. And no matter how else I tried to understand and share in her psychotherapy, I finally realized I had to go into therapy myself to *know.* I had visited Gelperin twice, once with Anne and once alone, not for myself but so that he would better understand our relationship. Now I found my own therapist and went to him once a week for several months.

The man was a fairly intelligent, rather kindly, middle-aged psychoanalyst, who seemed to have a good deal of integrity. I saw him religiously once a week—even when I slipped a disc to escape, then confronted the fact that this was *why* I'd slipped the disc, and literally crawled down to his office. I had already learned from Anne that there are *no* accidents. But after half a year about the only change for the better was in my lumbar, not lobe-al, region. And I *had* acquired a taste for peanut butter.

I fully realized that in a sense I was not a good candidate for therapy. By definition I did not have some pressing problem that was putting me in extreme pain. On the other hand, I virtually *always* have pressing problems that give me pain, this being the nature of my existence. And no area of my life has ever been problem-free, the positive end of the continuum inexorably bound to the negative. So in another sense I presented *more* material and possibilities for the therapist than the average patient.

After I left this analyst, still intensely involved with the therapeutic process because of Anne and my long-term fascination with psychology in general, the idea of this book was born. From then on, when I spoke with, heard of, or read about therapists or their patients, I was focused. When I saw a therapist for a few visits before beginning the actual writing of this book in early 1980, it was primarily I who had the clinical eye. Yes, I have my problems, problems I would very much like to get the better of. But I don't think they could be "cured" without "curing" also what it is that makes me tick.

There *are* valuable things therapy can do. Anne and I are the proof. Therapy has not cured my "problems," nor has it permanently cured Anne of the primary problem for which she went into therapy. Through its other benefits, however, therapy has enabled Anne to be a happier person more of the time, and this in turn has helped her handle many problems better, if not actually diminishing them. I think "sharing" her experience gave our relationship a further dimension. To Anne, of course, therapy supplied the strong but kind father she never knew. Also, because of her particular turn of mind, it gave her an activity she happens to love. Anne will keep going to her present therapist for as long as he lives, if for no other reason than the very good one that if she hadn't been a writer, she would have chosen to be a therapist. She assumes this role with many of her friends and acquaintances, and the role of "patient" is a perfect complement to it.

Yet the particular benefits she derived from therapy are uncommon. And the most important gift we both received can, I believe, be better gotten by *studying* therapy and psychology than by participating in it. That most important gain is *a better, fuller way of thinking*— which stems from a more profound recognition of the *subconscious* and an identification of the part it plays in our lives.

For those who have not studied psychology intimately or experienced some intensive therapy with a good doctor, no telling can substitute for that always growing, incredible *knowing* that comes from having "a handle" on that most magical part of you, called the subconscious. Often now when I miss a turnoff I know well when going to an appointment, I realize immediately that I should not be going or don't want to go there. And I stop and think why, and if the why is too convincing, I don't go. Now, when I am suddenly struck by a paranoia out of proportion to the situation, I know that I am really only placing my own anger onto something or someone else. This doesn't dissipate my anger, but it gives me an ultimate control over it. Now, I know hundreds of things like these —no, *thousands,* because a knowledge of psychology and psychoanalysis in particular has given me almost an instant understanding I never had of my behavior, my feelings, and of the behavior and feelings of others.

Knowing what Anne knows has been an invaluable tool. It has not fundamentally changed me. But it *has* immeasurably enlarged and deepened a dimension of myself, a singular dimension that allows me to view the same old Paul objectively for a moment, and to know in an instant what makes me tick.

Yet if I had been in intensive therapy for years, I *doubt* whether I would have that dimension. And the same old Paul would *not* be the same old Paul.

2
Therapy Needs Therapy

You may be a person who has never been in therapy, although you may have considered it.

You may be in therapy, know you're not getting enough out of it, and don't know whether you can get what you need from it, or how.

You may be an individual who is in therapy and feel it has helped you, but sense that unless you continue almost interminably, you'll feel that your crutches have suddenly been taken away and the leg is still broken.

Or it may be that someone close to you is in one of these situations.

Finally, it could be that you are a therapist, a man or woman who, on the one hand, is learned, intelligent, and "expert," and, on the other hand, has consistenly experienced the inability to help your patients enough, difficult though it is for you to face this fact.

Above all, you may be among the majority of us who must be our own therapists.

If this is a "how-to" book, it is because it may provide insights that you must make specifically meaningful. America pays great lip service to the fact that each of us is unique, with our own distinct set of capacities and past experiences, problems, and goals. The premise of *Same Time, Next Week?* is that infinite respect must be paid to each human being's uniqueness. The incessant flood of how-to books, with lists and rules on every hits-us-where-we-live subject, from making more money and performing better sexually to losing weight and getting rid of anxiety, persists precisely because in the long run they don't work except for the handful of readers who happen to be closely suited *as* individuals to the particular method of this-or-that particular book. For the other 99.99 percent the typical how-to book falsely offers a way to achieve what cannot be achieved by reading any how-to book.

Books are not the only "how-to" phenomenon in America. Therapy has become the biggest "how-to". Psychiatrists often adhere to rigid rules, or simply follow rigidly whatever "rules" they have happened upon. In actual fact, there are *no* rules in the field.

Same Time Next Week? does not deny that therapy can be a truly helpful and glorious experience. Nevertheless, there is no ignoring the disappointing reality that the overwhelming majority of psychiatrists and psychologists are not up to the task. Paul Meehl, former president of the American Psychological Association, who surveyed psychotherapists on the question of their colleagues' competency, discovered that "less than half, acutally closer to one-third or one-fourth of local practitioners" were thought by their colleagues to be worth recommending. And this by therapists themselves, in whose self-interest it is to uphold their profession.

Therapy, like brain surgery or oil painting, cannot be good for half an hour and then bad for half an hour. Because of this, therapy in America is doing much more harm than good.

This is not to say that psychotherapy is some singularly unsavory boondoggle. Much the same book as this could be written about stockbrokers or auto mechanics, attorneys or architects. With two differences. First, a lot has been said about the inefficiency or corruption of auto mechanics and attorneys. Second, if a therapist mishandles the engine of your psyche, you can't write off the loss and go down the street to have a part replaced.

It is therapy that needs its engine overhauled. Therapy in America . . . needs therapy.

3
The Ideal

Although a medical degree is required in order to become a psychiatrist, and a postgraduate university degree necessary to become a practicing psychologist, therapy is not a science and never will be. It is not in any facet a systematic discipline, nor can it be. Therapy is an art.

It is an art for which training can be somewhat helpful. Training can also be a strait jacket that needs to be untied and unlearned. In any event, a man or a woman cannot be trained to be a great therapist any more than a random individual can be trained to produce the works of a Van Gogh or a Leonardo da Vinci. Creating an ideal therapeutic relationship may be more difficult, in fact, since it involves not a blank canvas or a blank sheet of paper, but the opposite. The patient comes to the therapist as an infinitely complex puzzle, at some points maddeningly rigid, at others frustratingly ambiguous. Though he seldom grasps the solution at once, the therapist must almost immediately grasp the picture the puzzle will make. He must know which points are rigidly fixed and which ambiguities are lies or at least lies the patient is telling himself. The therapist must be unrelentingly objective, yet empathically human. The therapist, without allowing the patient to be dangerously dependent upon him, must, above all, make the patient *trust* him—and to do this the therapist must be the kind of person *outside* the office as well as inside who can be truly trusted.

And more. Much more.

There *are* therapists like this. There are Van Goghs and da Vincis, Dostoevskis and Hemingways, Edisons and Eisteins, Mme. Curies and Henry Thoreaus in psychiatry and psychology.

Such men and women, through the unique relationship they form with their patients, a relationship at times more intimate and more delicate than marriage, can give another human being

—tools for a new, more productive way of looking at things

—self-knowledge

—relief from pain

—a role model the patient did not have in childhood

—someone to whom the patient can truly talk, and someone who truly knows how to listen

—the catalyst to change for the better.

Such therapists exist. They are as rare as a da Vinci or an Einstein, and rightly so. There may be one in San Francisco and two more in London, but this does not mean there are many in Los Angeles or in New York. And if a person is fortunate enough to live where one of these artists practices therapy, how do you find *him* among the hundreds? Because of the nature of therapy, of the confidentiality of the relationship, the giants in this field are not known by reputation.

Most of all, if you would search for such a therapist, how do you avoid becoming the patient of one who is less? For here, less is not more. The painting of a technically excellent, intelligent, but unoriginal artist—an excellent copy of a copy, in other words—may be worth a fair price in a gallery, but is virtually worthless in therapy. The work of an undisciplined young painter showing great promise may be worth nurturing, purchasing, and putting away for a few years. In therapy promise is nothing next to performance, and you cannot "put away" a therapist who *some day* may be fine. The dime-store painting of a hack may be worth hanging in an out-of-the-way bathroom, but monstrously disturbing if hung in an out-of-the-way room of your mind. A talented but flawed writer may produce one or two good books and a dozen inconsistent or bad books. Yet the *totality* of the therapist is channeled into *each* therapeutic relationship, and if there are even one or two "bad books" within him, or even some only fair ones, that level will ultimately be the touchstone for his therapeutic relationships. A well-paid accountant may make a handful of mistakes in a week; a handful of mistakes each week for a therapist is disastrous to his patients.

There *are* ideal therapists. This does not mean they are perfect; it means that their imperfections, even when apparent, are under such control that they virtually never run counter to the artistry of the therapeutic relationship. All the others will mistake some of the rigid points of a psychic pattern for malleable, ambiguous areas of the personality. They will, at critical times, lack objectivity or empathy. They will, if unwittingly, encourage the patient's dependence upon them and, in the same proportion, lose the patient's trust. They will seem to hold the answers to everything, but the solutions to next to nothing. They will turn out patients who know more that is worth less. Better no therapy than this kind of therapy. The terrorizing tumult of a human psyche that has been well-meaningly sabotaged is invisible and silent, but no less a tragedy.

The tragedy is inevitable when the therapist is less than an artist—is himself still searching for tools toward a new way of thinking, still in need of crucial self-knowledge and of his own pain being relieved, still desperately attempting to be a model *he* has never had and in need of the relationship with the patient. And . . . simply not happy, yearning to change for the better himself.

Obviously, there is not a Grand Canyon but a continuum between the therapist who, though pretty good, isn't good enough and the therapist who is a great artist at what he does. Even greatness can err, and someone whose median is pretty good will once in a while be very good. But, again, two things cannot be emphasized too strongly: (1) The longer the therapy goes on, the lower the batting average of the fairly good therapist becomes. (2) Therapy is a unique field where any batting average with a patient less than near perfect is strictly minor league. Nor is the possibility of making up for an error likely. The therapeutic relationship is *not* a baseball game, nor a not-too-bad hammering out of a dent on your fender or an attorney who charged you too much and then didn't get you out of the traffic ticket.

Therapy is a building in which you will eventually live, a house that must be constructed from the ground up. Lay the foundation inexpertly, and the house will sink and crumble and be more dangerous than no house at all, no matter how beautiful or clear the temporary view from the picture window in the living room.

4
Our New National Religion – Therapy

Remember when there weren't enough doctors to go around (an excess of physicians and therapists is predicted by 1990), but they made house calls?

Remember when the priest or minister or rabbi was something of a personal friend, to whom you could tell your troubles without going to confession, or whose temple your children could visit on the high holidays without a $900 pledge to the building fund?

Remember when a neighbor could *really* be depended upon? Or you *knew* your neighbors? Or when there was an older member of your family close by to whom you could always go for advice and help? Or when your pastor or rabbi was interested in *you* rather than in fund raising or social progress?

These were our therapists. The family physician—the

family physician—who would come to your house, see you in your primary environment and treat the total patient, usually performed therapy beautifully, no more than a handful of times a year.

No longer.

Some of us still love and respect our fathers, though at times it is boggling how few do, but virtually never does the family father hold final respect as an empathic but knowing authority figure—any more than George Washington does. Many of us are still deeply religious and respect the magistrates of the church and temple, but they are no longer magistrates of our therapy. Nor is the busy doctor. Even if he weren't so busy, in a world where almost all physical pain can be banished as quickly as TV commercials proclaim, emotional pain stands out in bold relief, and the specialists have taken over. The therapist moved into a vacuum, and the first question is whether he belongs there.

The evidence strongly suggests that if we cannot today go to our parents, preachers, friends, close relatives, or neighbors for therapy, then neither should we generally go to therapists for it. The 17.8 million Americans who spent $23 billion last year for their mental health aren't getting what they paid for. Therapy may not only be a bad buy, it can be destructive. Several years ago, *U.S. News & World Report* stated: "Our nation's 27,000 psychiatrists and innumerable therapists at other levels find their credibility and effectiveness being questioned more sharply than ever." More and more the cultural caricaturization of the therapist has deteriorated from the Freud-like analyst to the psychiatrist of the recent movie *Serial,* who, between snorts of cocaine, informs a ten-year-old patient that the boy needs to get in touch with what he wanted as a child.

Nevertheless, we go to therapists in greater droves then ever. Many companies now have therapists on their staffs, as do our community organizations and, of course, the federal government, which, one way or another, is allocating so much money toward mental health that we are becoming the land of the free and the home of the analyzed. Moreover, government's cretinish inability to run either itself or the country has only widened the vacuum of cultural leadership and allowed therapy an even greater primacy. And yet, though therapy is now middle-aged, flabby, and not able to do the job, it continues to influence our lives, directly or indirectly. Don't say that because you have never seen a therapist and don't intend to see one, and know a lot of people of the same persuasion, therapy has not touched you. It has *more* than touched everything important in America. It plays perfectly into both our political modes—the brother's keeper —the Judeo-Christian ethic of the conservatively oriented, and the government-as-keeper morality of the liberal. Through the proliferating use of "insanity" as a measure for serious crime, the testimony of therapists has become pivotal to our system of so-called justice. It has taken over the market research that generates our television programs and determines the commercials to pay for them. We decry the moronic manipulativeness of the media; we bemoan the killers and rapists who walk among us because some therapist has testified that they weren't in their right minds when committing the crimes!

"The world is sick," we say. And the implication? The world needs *more* therapy. Actually, it may be therapy, and our attitude toward it, that is sick.

5
Believe It or Not, Therapists Are Like Us

The thirty-three-year-old woman walks into the therapist's office, and what does she encounter?

She sees a forty-five-year-old man who is highly intelligent, willing to listen to her in a way her husband seldom does, and, above all, a professional in the field of solving problems. She sees a purported professional. She may even see the closest thing to a god.

A middle-aged man enters the office of a therapist who is dressed casually but well, with a beard that adds further to his seeming maturity. He looks to be the fountain of wisdom, of empathy.

A young mother faces a handsome psychologist with a dazzling reputation. She sees someone attractive to her in a way that no other man can be. She sees a miracle worker.

These patients no doubt have problems. But by far their biggest problem from the moment they walk into the doctor's office is that what they *wish* the therapist to be is how they see him. Now and then the therapist may not fall too far short of their expectations. Much more often, he will. Yet they will continue to misperceive him for precisely the same reason they are visiting him: Viewing him as a god or a miracle worker or, at the very least, an extremely wise and good man *temporarily relieves their pain.*

But the therapist is not a god or a miracle worker and is seldom a surpassingly good or wise man. In fact, he or she is someone, all in all, pretty much like you and me. Some try to be good and succeed. Some try to be good and don't succeed. And many don't try to be good at all. A friend of mine who is a partner in a major brokerage firm (and who possesses such integrity that often when I have called him and asked him what to buy, he answers, "Nothing right now"), made this observation: "Stockbrokers are the same as any other profession. Eighty percent are incompetent. Of the remaining twenty percent, most are only fair. One or two percent actually do the job the way it should be done."

Whatever the true percentage among therapists of competents, hangers-on, and incompetents, the crucial difference between therapy and virtually any other profession must be reemphasized. If your stockbroker gives you several tips and you lose money, your stockbroker will lose you. If you go to a therapist and you become worse, you may feel that you need him even more. The very fact that mental and emotional stability is what we are seeking from the therapist tends to make us feel unqualified to judge his results squarely. But who is going to judge him?

So people continue with the wrong therapists, or with therapists who are wrong for therapy. The patients don't change for the better, and certainly the therapists don't. No matter how dubious their results, they continue to do business at the same old stand, usually with the same old customers and/or referrals from those customers.

I entered Haverford, a small college with a good reputation, in 1953. More than half of the freshmen intended to be doctors. By their sophomore or junior years, thank goodness, some had decided not to go into medicine. Yet a majority continued on and became physicians or therapists.

Out of a freshman class of about 120 I recall a few who combined enough dedication, empathy, and intelligence for me to trust them with my physical health, let alone my mental health. Most went into another field. Far more disturbing than this loss, though, was that we didn't lose the rest. I clearly recall the opening weeks on campus, mingling with the other freshmen before I knew why they were there. They were your average "above average" group. Some were very bright, most weren't. Most were insecure, some weren't. Some were very ambitious, many fairly ambitious, others unambitious. Many were a number were short, a lot of them in between. I could see more than half of them making good administrators, businessmen, career diplomats, lawyers, social workers, and deans of Haverford or some other college, but I could not see even a handful holding lives—or the human psyche—in their hands. I was no different than they were. And I would not now, or then presume to help others as a life's work. One upperclassman I particularly liked had decided to be a psychiatrist early on. He had a fetching personality and was a good listener, with piercing gray eyes that seemed to understand everything in lieu of his not saying too much of anything. One Sunday morning, though, he did say something very specific: He told me I had danced too close with Anne (we were to be married a few months later) and should watch myself if I cared what people thought. That was the end of our friendship. I didn't care what people thought—particularly people like him.

No doubt he matured later?

The essential answer to that question is best revealed in a chance meeting I had a few years ago with another pre-med I knew from the University of Chicago, which I attended prior to Haverford. He was a good fellow, from another part of the country, not unintelligent but simply, by interest or the fabric of his personality, not at all suited to being a therapist. I had thought of him now and then in the more than twenty years since college, masochistically wondering what it would be like to be a patient of his. Lo and behold, I was having coffee in a suburban Chicago restaurant one day when he recognized me and said hello. Ordinarily not one for reunions, accidental or otherwise, I found myself impelled to make small talk with him for a minute or two in order to ask the big question, "Well, what are you doing here? Why aren't you treating patients in Florida?"

"Oh, I didn't become a psychiatrist," he replied. "I'm in advertising."

A colossal feeling of relief swept over me.

But I don't feel relief when I receive the alumni bulletin and find out how many are practicing medicine or therapy. Many of those to whom I have spoken don't much want to do what they are doing. And I have seldom known anyone to be really good at something he doesn't enjoy, and this becomes truer as the years pass. However, the money, the prestige, the security, the power lure too many young men and women into the field of medicine in general and therapy in particular, which is obviously why we are on the verge of a great doctor glut. One therapist poignantly confided in me, "I always wanted to be an architect." But he was pushed along for most of the usual reasons toward medical school and, finding himself over the age of thirty, when it would have seemed ridiculous to throw away a dozen years of expensive training, he of course opened an office and the practice of psychotherapy. Like so many other therapists, he is either divorced or not that happily married, is sometimes plagued by

bothersome physical problems, from overweight to hemorrhoids, masturbates to his sexual fantasies of movie
stars and his own patients, is extremely susceptible to
praise, and all the rest of it. Therapists generally take long
and frequent vacations to get away from their job, but
seldom change their line of work. Unlike most of us, economic conditions seldom force them into another field.
And, like most of us, even though they may not be too
happy with what they do, they are resistant to change.

And *we* are resistant—to changing therapists, to leaving therapy. One reason is that, like cigarettes, it is a
difficult habit to break. As was said recently in the American Psychoanalytic Association's own journal, there is a
basic narcissistic pleasure for the patient in the therapeutic situation. Most of us spend much of our lives trying to
get a word in edgewise. When we do, the listener usually
isn't that attentive to what we have to say. When we go
into therapy, we feel sure there is someone who cares. We
pay him to care.

But there's something else. The therapist does possess
a manner that is different from ours, a manner that tends
to throw us off-balance and make us feel he knows something we don't. Every once in a while in life you meet
someone with this manner, and you feel the same way.
But virtually every therapist has it, because it is indige-
nous to the profession. It is the manner of a scrupulous
listener and observer. There is no small talk with a therapist, for he knows that the smallest remark of yours is

meaningful, and, if nothing else, he is trained to look for that meaning. He will not interrupt you; he will not even be *waiting* to interrupt you, as most everyone else is. Tell him something that does not require an answer, even while bumping into him on the street, and he won't give one. Or if an answer is required, if you ask a therapist what's new, for example, he will not answer with the peremptory, "Nothing. What's new with you?" Something is always new.

This disarming approach does indeed disarm us. Our daily relationships are lubricated by an amalgam of half-truths that supposedly pass without question. The therapist deals in literal meanings. He forces us to take off our verbal masks. But . . . that does not mean he has removed *his.*

As if it weren't enough that we revere our doctors and therapists in particular as demigods because they deal with physical and psychic health, as if it weren't enough that we often envy them on a human level because they are respected by our society for their education and income, their manner—which is almost automatic after long years of training—leads us to have faith in their wisdom and objectivity.

But again, except for that disarming manner, they are pretty much like the rest of us. They make mistakes. They have problems. And, as a matter of fact, they may have *more* problems and make *more* mistakes than you and I. In a Knight Newspaper Syndicate story not long ago enti-

tled "Therapy For Therapists—It Shows They're Human"
it was reported that "psychologists and psychiatrists esti-
mate that one-third to one-half of all mental health profes-
sionals undergo psychotherapy at some point. For the
general population, surveys find that the proportion is
much lower."

Most therapists would answer this by saying that they
above all know the value of therapy, and this is why they
themselves seek it more than other people. The simple
fact is that therapists may need therapy more than the
rest of us.

6
The Cowardly Therapist

He usually awakens about the same time as the rest of us. Next to him will be a wife he might or might not love, quite possibly his second wife. The sounds of children awakening for school, unless they are grown and have left home, are in the background. Though he generally lives in an expensive house or apartment, there may be one bathroom too few, and he might have to wait or rush. If he's on a diet or a little late, he'll catch a cup of coffee near the office (unless his office is at home). In his briefcase, if he tries to keep up with his field, are some articles he means to read, as well as bills to pay and other mail. In the coffee shop he notices how attractive the new waitress is, but he puts that aside when his son's drug problem comes to mind. As he rises to leave, he feels a twinge in his ribs. Nothing to worry about—coronary pain is higher up—but he worries anyway. He hasn't been getting enough exercise.He purchases a paper, skims the headlines. Problems. Problems. *Problems.*

When he enters his office, he feels the same thing most of the rest of us do when we get to work each day: The one thing we don't need is . . . more problems.

Yet the therapist makes his living through other people's problems. He's damn glad they have them and glad they bring them to *him.*

With reservations.

Is the fellow at 10:15 a borderline psychotic and dangerous—to the therapist?

Is the woman at 1:00 as attractive as the waitress in the restaurant, more educated, and falling in love with him?

Is he too emotionally involved with the fifteen-year-old boy at 3:40 who has a drug problem very similar to his son's?

One of comedian Mel Brooks' most insightful sketches revolves around a quasi-therapist, who, when a disturbed woman is ushered into his office, begins screaming and shouting to his nurse to get her out because she's sick, sick, sick! We laugh, since it seems almost unthinkable that a therapist would feel this. Yet Shakespeare wisely told us that truth is spoken in jest, and Freud flatly stated that there are no "jokes." Every therapist is confronted consistently by people who may be dangerous to him in one way or another. Or personally disgusting. Or boring.

The Dark Mirror, a farsighted motion picture of the

mid-forties, in which Olivia de Havilland played a schizophrenic twin who murdered several men and attempted
to do the same with her sister and her psychiatrist, cannot
be dismissed. How can a therapist *not* think of this each
time a new patient enters the office? How many therapists
have been called in the middle of the night by suicidal
patients or in the middle of dinner for "crisis" anxiety
attacks and depressions? Or that frantic call or banging on
the door may be the patient's mate, lover, parent, child.

Or the devoted patient, when the therapist will go only
so far in the relationship, may suddenly turn hateful and
one day be sitting not in the therapist's office but in a
lawyer's office drawing up a malpractice suit against the
shrink. A recent *Chicago Sun-Times* article entitled "Patients Don't Shrink From Suing Analysts" reveals that
malpractice suits against therapists are showing a dra-
matic increase every year. Whereas malpractice suits
against psychiatrists and psychologists were once rare, in
Chicago and Cook County alone they are nearly doubling
annually. Moreover, the *type* of suit against therapists has
changed. It used to be that an individual usually sued only
if the therapist seemed a charlatan—such as promising
the patient a complete cure for his alcoholism or homosexuality or some equally extreme syndrome. Now patients are suing for just about anything that doesn't come
out right or fails to please them. And in an alarming number of cases the therapists are losing.

When a psychiatrist sits down at the dinner table, the

last thing he wants is an emergency phone call or a sub-poena. It's difficult enough for him to handle his own problems at home. Because of all this, most therapists do not want to jeopardize their good income, their good rep-utation, nor their security and safety, by fooling around with people who have *real* problems. Would *you* if you were in their shoes?

But if safety first is the most profitable policy personally for the therapist, it is not necessarily the best way to go for the patient. Those who *seem* seriously ill are too often hospitalized, not for their own good, but for the thera-pist's good. Many of these people need out-patient psy-chotherapy only; the therapist is often "too busy" to work them in, however. They eventually end up with less quali-fied therapists, who may do them more harm than good.

In view of these considerations, the majority of thera-pists try to stick to the "average" individual with "aver-age" neuroses. The individual may improve somewhat through treatment, simply because *any* kind of psychic self-examination would result in improvement. Like a new weight-loss regimen, though, the initial support and improvement soon diminish to the point of almost no return. Still, as there have been some positive results, the patient may keep going. And going. And the therapist seldom argues with this at all, implicitly holding out hope to his clients that there will be further improvement at some time or another. Thus, unfortunately, there is often an inverse ratio between how rational a therapist is and how he uses that rationality within his work. He gravitates toward the "safer" patients, and plays it safe with them. Because a shrink can probe into virtually anyone's psyche and upset it if he so chooses, the last thing most shrinks want is to see a patient leave their office in a state of anxiety or of depression, even if that is the price that must be paid for less anxiety and fewer depressions in the future.

In a word, many therapists—precisely because they *are* like most other people—take the coward's way. And for those who would risk now and then, for the sake of truth and integrity, the kind of treatment they realize is needed, the ever-present specter hanging over their heads of our supralegal society cautions "be prudent, hold off."

Hold off healing.

7
The Sick Therapist

Too many therapists, however, far from being cowardly, take more than rational risks with their patients. They take big, irrational gambles. They do it because they themselves are in far more trouble than the patient.

A recent study by the Pennsylvania Welfare Department, for example, revealed that fully two-thirds of the psychiatrists at some of the state's mental hospitals were suffering from "serious mental illness". Stunning as that percentage is, many other facts bear it out. Evidence is difficult to obtain for therapists in private practice, but, again, the figures for therapists who are sicker than their patients is alarmingly high. Psychologist Dr. Pamela K. S. Patrick made a study revealing that those who work with physically and emotionally ill people have the highest "burn out" rate of any profession. The question this and other similar studies has not answered is: To what degree does practicing therapy make therapists sick, or do people with incipient mental or emotional illness tend to become therapists in the first place?

The grim irony here, of course, is that a major premise of psychology would tell us that indeed those people with a particular kind of emotional disturbance gravitate to jobs in which they feel least alien, though for which they are not necessarily well-suited. Too many teachers are people who feel an inherent powerlessness, possibly from an unfortunate childhood situation, and thus enter a field where they are the only adult among power-limited youngsters. Many violent personalities wind up in the military or on the police force, because violence is their *de rigeur*. By the same token, a lot of intelligent, educated young men and women who sense that they are emotionally sick, rather than becoming patients, become the "doctors." The role itself gives them a guise of health. And the very fact that they are with the emotionally disturbed makes them feel comfortable. They are more at home in a world of mental illness.

I observed one psychiatrist a few years ago (and I could make much the same observation about many) who appeared extremely disturbed. He had two unsuccessful marriages behind him, partly because he had not been able to perform sexually; his children were already quite fouled up before adolescence; and he was given to frequent breakdowns. He had seen more than one therapist for his problems, to no avail. He suffered a nervous facial twitch that was very disconcerting. His patients almost all became worse for therapy with him–those, that is, who stayed on more than a few months. However, as is the case with most psychiatrists, new patients would inevitably replace them, so he had the typical lucrative practice. More than one of his patients attempted suicide. Still, the therapist he himself was seeing did not advise him to leave the profession, out of fear of recrimination. And also, as therapy is so deuces-wild, it ill behooves all but the best therapists to take an absolute stand on anything related to the human psyche.

In all fairness, I recall a psychologist who did leave the field voluntarily. Unable to help his patients on a one-to-one basis (and honest enough to face that fact), he stopped seeing people privately and instead held therapy groups and encounter weekends. They, too, proved so unproductive that finally the man gave up the practice of therapy completely and went into business with a relative. "I was kidding myself," he said. "I wasn't helping anybody. I really wasn't qualified to be a therapist, even though I had gone through all the training and have a high I.Q. In all candor, I was doing more harm than good. I'm seeing a therapist now, but even if I improve, I surely don't feel qualified to treat people again."

Once again, it cannot be emphasized enough that even if the rate of mental illness and related incompetency among therapists were the same instead of higher, than for the general population, it would be soberingly significant. The therapist is involved in the kind of work where he must have his own problems under control in order to help others control their problems. The GP who is troubled by a crumbling marriage or a youngster on drugs may not relate as well to his patients, but he can still adequately read an X-ray or interpret a blood count. The therapist with problems may be compared more to the surgeon with an unsteady hand from Parkinson's disease.

There are all sorts of reasons that practicing therapy can threaten one's mental balance. The most important, and one about which the therapist can do nothing, is that he or she is often *attempting to do the impossible.* There is a real question whether therapy can "work" at all, or if, rather than a method for human improvement, it is, as Freud told us, mainly a tool for investigating human behavior. If Freud was right, this would certainly explain the many patients who emerge from therapy no better. But what about those who go into therapy and come out feeling better or doing better, sometimes with therapists who are sick?

It could be that the patient would have gotten better anyway. The well-known British psychologist, Hans J. Eysenck, undertook an intensive study on the effects of psychotherapy (his report published in the January 1965 issue of the *International Journal of Psychiatry*). Groups of similar cases were compared over an extended period: one group of those who had been treated psychotherapeutically; another with chemical or physical means, but primarily with the age-old prescription of rest or recuperation in clinics or convalescent homes; and finally those whose illness was diagnosed but not treated. The primary conclusion of this study was that the number of major improvements among untreated neurotics was equal to that among those who had received any form of therapy. The brain is an organ composed of cells just as are the lungs and the kidneys, and except where the illness is terminal and the body's immunological system is no longer effective, the inexorable thrust of the human mechanism is toward self-healing, health, and survival.

Another possibility is that the patient is *not* feeling or doing better, but has been *convinced* that he is. This is a dangerous line of inquiry, for who among us has the right to tell you or me that we are *not* happy and more productive if *we* think we are? It is arguable that one man's productivity is another man's problem, one woman's happiness another woman's horror. Nevertheless, many of us, through the therapist, sell ourselves a bill of goods about how happy or meaningful we are, or believe ourselves to be, as a defense against the pain of confronting what we truly are and truly want.

One thing is certain: Mental illness, even emotional instability, in a therapist is extremely dangerous to the patient. Though mental illness or emotional instability in anyone is obviously a disadvantage, in the therapist it is hazardous. The secretary with a progressing psychological problem may turn out sloppy letters, an editor may miss deadlines. But they also may not. For all of us have neuroses, but we can often dichotomize ourselves to a point where our work and even personal responsibilities are not affected. Many human beings, as Freud first recognized, sublimate their sicknesses into their work or into their relationships and are more productive or charismatic because of it. The therapist is *not*. If he is sick or disturbed, he will produce a sicker or more disturbed patient. The reason is self-evident: It is precisely sickness and disturbance he is treating.

Second, if the secretary composes a sloppy letter to a particular client, her boss will probably monitor it and attempt to make things right. Moreover, he can protect himself in the future, if enough sloppy letters are sent out, by terminating her employment. With the therapist, there is no monitor. Moreover, if his psyche is in chaos, he doesn't merely write one "sloppy letter" to his patient, but many, week upon week, possibly year upon year.

It may be said that the patient can terminate with the therapist just as the boss can fire the secretary or the secretary can leave that job for a better one. *Seldom.*

The patient who is having problems finds it difficult to get up and leave. Or if she or he does, it is to find a better therapist, and it is hard to find one. For the new therapist starts at a disadvantage. He does not have the rapport with, or the knowledge of the patient that the former therapist did. The patient cannot immediately refer to

43

intimate things that matter and expect a new man to understand. Also, the less competent and more emotionally unstable the therapist, the less he will want a patient to leave. And the therapist has tremendous influence, to say the least, in this matter.

Even if a patient does want to leave, even if a therapist is not sick and not incompetent and feels it probably advisable to discontinue their sessions, the biggest obstacle to termination is that ... *there really is no such thing at present as termination in the field of therapy.*

8
Same Time Next Week?
Therapy and Endless Illness

A former patient tells this story:

"I was divorced in 1975, left with the care of my two children and only a small amount of child support. I started to pursue my former career of commercial artist, something I had wanted to do for years, and eventually moved to a position with loads of opportunity. My only superior was a woman a few years older than myself who was going through a bad marital breakup, but this didn't seem to impede her work, and I thought I had an ideal job.

"I'd been in therapy for almost three years. My psychologist, an obviously brilliant man, in his late forties with a top reputation, had aided me through my own divorce, helped me to see that it was inevitable and that I could function on my own and possibly find much more happiness than I had known before. I think I could have gotten along without him, but I was grateful as hell for him, had really come to think of him as close to perfect as anyone could be. I knew, of course, that he was human. But in our sessions each week, whatever faults he had never seemed to show themselves.

"After the first year of therapy, for financial reasons, and also because I felt I could make it on my own, I brought up the matter of leaving him. He handled it pretty much as he handled everything else, except that I had the gnawing feeling that *he didn't want me to.* It was the first time I didn't feel quite right about what was going on between us, but I had so much faith in him that I stayed. After a few more months, I really did feel like leaving him and brought it up again. 'If you think you're ready,' was his response.

"Well, I felt I was ready or I wouldn't have brought it up. But I could tell *he* didn't think I was ready. It was all so subtle, though, that I couldn't bring it out in the open. If I had said to him at that point, 'You don't seem to feel I am ready to leave,' he would have answered that he didn't say that. Anyway, before the end of that session, he did something he had never done before: He brought up something that had always bothered me, but not a great deal. It was one of those problems you can live with, though you'd rather not have it, of course. We began discussing it, kept discussing it the next week and the next, and before long my leaving wasn't an issue anymore.

"That happened more than once. Seven months later I

was bound and determined to leave therapy, when he brought up something else I had mentioned a long time ago that he knew bothered me. But it also wasn't of major consequence. Still, once we got into it, it assumed more importance. And another bunch of months passed while we talked about it and whatever else came up in my life. There's a big difference between a therapist saying, if *you* think you're ready and his saying '*Yes,* I think you're about ready.'

"So I stayed. And stayed. I can see now that I should have left, and that it was something in *him,* not *me,* that was keeping me there. Sure, I had other problems. Who doesn't? But there just wasn't that much going on in my sessions with him anymore. I was there only to keep the relationship with him going, and, when a man helps you, particularly a therapist, there's a strong pull to keep that relationship going, so it wasn't as if I marched in every time and said, 'I'm leaving!'

"By the third year there were times I felt like doing that. Once I'd get in there, though, I couldn't feel that angry at someone who had helped me so much. And you always wonder in the back of your mind whether the therapist doesn't know something you don't know— you're sure he does. Eventually the day came when *I* knew that no matter how good a therapist he was or how knowledgeable he was, I was spinning my wheels there and spending money that could have been better used in my life. I simply blurted out that I wanted to leave after the following week; I didn't feel I could get up and end week; I didn't feel I could get up and end it right there that same day, after three years. Once I said that, he acted out of character for the first time. He said okay, then let's see if we can't get all our work done in the rest of this session and the next. In fact, he said he thought I ought to come one more time that week and twice the next so we could be sure to get everything done. I was so glad he was going along with ending things that I agreed. But I'll be damned if those two sessions a week didn't go on for three months. He just had a way of keeping it going.

"I had to leave by writing him a letter. It sounds ridiculous to say it, but it was the only way I could do it at the time. The second to last week I actually flat out said that the next session would be the last, and I'll never forget his words: 'I really don't think you're quite ready yet. Why don't we go a few more sessions and then we'll talk about termination.' *The man wouldn't let me go.*

"So the day after one Thursday session I drove all the way back later and put a note under his door when I knew he was through for the day. I told him how much I appreciated what he had done for me, but felt I could live my life without therapy now. And so on. Nothing happened for about three months, and then he called me to ask how I was doing. Before I knew it, we had talked fifteen minutes and I had told him a couple of things that were bothering me at the time—is life ever perfect?—and he suggested I come in. It was plain he wanted me back as a patient, whether I needed it or not. I told him I'd like to try and work these things out myself, that they really weren't disturbing me very much, but that I'd call him in a week or two if I did need the appointment. I never called him. But he's called me several times since, and the same thing goes on every time. He's a good therapist, but he just doesn't want to let a patient go, and that's his failing. I can imagine that a less strong-minded person than myself would never get out of his office."

This former patient's observation about few people being able to leave their therapist is true. That she did so is an exception. But her therapist isn't really the exception, as far as termination is concerned. *Most therapists don't want their patients to terminate, discourage their patients from terminating, or, even when they think termination of therapy is advisable, don't know how to go about it.*

I asked one therapist, a respected, older man in the field, these two questions: (1) What percentage of the time do you bring up terminating therapy with a patient? and (2) What would you say is known about termination within your field generally? He answered; (1) "I honestly never have suggested termination," and (2) "Hardly anything is known in our field about termination. We don't really know anything about it."

Though there are a minority of therapists who do urge a patient to terminate and have their own particular method of doing so, *most don't.* Termination—the rational, mutually agreed upon ending of psychotherapy—is rare.

Why? For a variety of personal reasons and for the professional reason that *there simply is no real definitive methodology in the field of psychiatry or psychology for ending the therapeutic relationship.*

The literature in the psychiatric and psychological journals on this aspect of therapy is astonishly meager. What literature there is usually turns out at best to be no more than common sense, and usually much less. Let's look for example, at an article in *The American Journal of Psychotherapy,* October 1979, by Drs. Leonard Maholick and Don Turner, entitled "Termination: That Difficult Farewell." The authors' experience with the literature in group termination parallels the sparcity of it for one-to-one ending of therapy: "We have noted how little has been written in the professional literature on the nature and the clinical management of good termination." They then proceed to indicate the proper *times* for termination: (1) when there is an actual contract that has concluded; (2) "when the patient in the group has progressed as far as he wants"; (3) "when terminations are precipitated by unexpected developments such as job changes . . . and financial reverses"; (4) when the patient does such things as "flagrant and recurring abusive attacking of others" or "refusal to pay his bill"; (5) "When the patient becomes psychotic"; and a couple of others along similar lines.

Frankly, this is one of the more sensible articles on the subject (and by two men of excellent standing in the field) and thus points out in even bolder relief how little is really definitively understood about this problem. Of *course* it is time for termination when a patient becomes psychotic or the contract period is over or the patient moves to another city. The real issue, the *only* issue, is: Within an ordinary, fair relationship between therapist and patient devoid of stonewalling outside or inside events, how soon and when is the patient in an effective position to carry on for himself, and *how* is this determined?

Hilliard Levinson, in private practice as well as supervisor of the Illinois Children's Home and Aid Society in Evanston, puts it more aptly in an article about him in *Human Behavior* entitled "The Last Session: It Can Be Traumatic": The termination phase of therapy, which he [Levinson] prefers to be extended rather than abrupt, should be like a musical coda summarizing the themes and motifs that precede it. These final measures, he says, will usually contain some grief and mourning about the loss, perhaps even anxiety, but also contentment and joy at the therapeutic goals it achieved.

This is a beautiful statement of what termination should be like, but nowhere in personal interviews or in the literature of the field have I been able to find evidence that even a meaningful minority of therapists have a handle on the composition of the final movement of such a symphony.

I have known patients who have become clearly worse after having gone into therapy, but whose therapists tell them that this is the necessary storm before the calm. I have known patients to become clearly the better for therapy—until they try to leave their therapists. Then all their problems and more return, the sure sign the therapy was unsuccessful. Freud did not write *Analysis: Terminable and Interminable* as a lark.

What does this mean to *you?* Whether you are in therapy now, have been in it but are presently not seeing a therapist, or contemplating therapy in the future—or know and care about somebody who is—the problem of termination within the profession is in itself enough to weigh against successful therapy. What should, what *must*, be a finite, goal-oriented relationship from the outset is instead an ambiguous, often endless dependency. A minority of therapists are predisposed to termination; a minority of that minority are operably knowledgeable about it.

And where there is no meaningful termination target, there can also be no success in the therapy. If you can never rationally, autonomously leave your therapist, or he never wants you to leave, what kind of treatment is that? Therapy then becomes not really regular outpatient visits to the doctor, but, in a deeper sense, incarceration in a psychoanalytic nursing home with extended leaves of absence.

Yet if nontermination-targeted therapy is almost always gapingly negative, therapy leading purposefully toward termination has these positive values: (1) It can end therapy sooner and better, allowing the patient to use the tools himself that therapy has given. (2) It almost automatically creates a structure that is more productive. (3) It sets up a standard by which both patient *and therapist* can be measured.

And there is still another value: Therapy built upon as early and rational an ending as possible is a *model.*

Let's say you go to a therapist to learn how to deal better with your mother-in-law. A lot of people have problems with their mother-in-law, but, say, she lives with you, she's very dear to your wife, but is a crusty, domineering woman who consistently creates trouble. A good therapist can aid you with this situation by helping you to understand it and see alternatives. Possibly she should not live with you, and as a result of therapy, you will be equipped to show that to your wife and then to her mother. Possibly she has to keep living in your home, but on somewhat different terms, guided by a different set of reactions you will have after successful therapy. But once you do know how to deal with the problem, you should not keep going to the therapist about it. It is your problem, you know what to do about it, and it is up to you to handle it. It is no longer the therapist's problem unless he *wants* it to be *his* problem. And the therapist should not want this.

Still, a majority of therapeutic relationships do end, don't they?

The answer is that they *end,* but they do not *terminate.* They do not finish with therapeutic success. Sure, many people go for only a few months, others for a few years, after which they decide to leave for their own reasons. But the point is that the patient *leaves*, he does not terminate therapy. He may have gained some insight about himself, but only some. Possibly a lot of these people will return to their therapists at a later date, or to some other therapist and go through the same experience again—an incomplete experience, an aborted relationship. Indeed, *this* might be the problem in their lives for which they went to the therapist in the first place.

Finally, there is the patient who is not a patient—the woman or man who disavows the same time, next week game. He or she may visit a therapist only a few times, or not at all. This person sees at the outset, or senses from those he knows who have been in therapy, that what he will be embarking on is not a road leading somewhere, but an ever circling maze.

What can have no meaningful ending should never have had a beginning.

9
The Art of Termination

Proper termination in therapy is up to *you.*

Ideally, it is the therapist's responsibility, but it is a responsibility most therapists have disavowed.

If the therapist resists your attempts to participate in structuring your therapy about termination, and does not substitute an equally viable termination "schedule," this may be a clue that he is the wrong therapist for you—or for almost anybody.

How do you go about preparing for a successful ending of therapy from the outset?

First, there *are* patients who should *not* terminate, or at least think about termination for some time. They are a small, a very small minority. They fall into two groups: (1) those whose problems are so deep and complex that intensive psychoanalysis or, at least, long-term therapy is a necessity; such patients should not even begin to think of ending therapy until it has been a demonstrable success, with a consistently more positive emotional outlook and behavior to match, and (2) those infrequent "patients," such as my wife, to whom therapy is part of a way of life.

Anne loves the *process* of therapy, much as a dedicated scientist loves his laboratory, or a school child loves a "free period." So often, with the one or two therapists who have been right for her, she has burst into the house after a session saying, "It's wonderful! Wonderful," like someone who has just seen an exhilarating movie. She no longer really goes to "cure" her "problems," nor to learn a better way of thinking. She goes because she likes, *loves,* participating in the process of therapy.

But this *is* the exception, because Anne has simply made therapy one of the few major activities of her life, engaging in it as both therapy and "therapist," reading about it, writing about it, living it. Though it most certainly helped her in a strictly therapeutic way with Gelperin, now it "helps" her more in Freud's way: as a tool for understanding the human mind.

I also have an acquaintance who grew up in what can only be termed a psychotic environment. Two of the four children are institutionalized, a third, though in his early forties, still lives with his parents. My acquaintance would probably be in an institution were it not for seeing a therapist twice weekly. As it is, much of the time he is on the borderline of a breakdown, but only once or twice has gone over that line. Before therapy, he could not hold a job, experienced long periods of depression when he had to be taken care of, and had virtually no solid relationships. I don't know how good his therapist is—what I've been told leads me to believe that my friend could do better—but simply visiting an adequate therapist twice weekly is evidently enough to enable this man to function. He might function better with a better therapist, but I seriously doubt he could ever get along without therapy.

Such special cases notwithstanding, termination of therapy is proper, desirable, and necessary.

And it should be the *first* concern when the patient begins a relationship with the therapist. How? Ask. Spend a session or two explaining to the therapist why you are there, but keep in mind that you're interviewing *him.* Discuss the different scenarios he might see for dealing with what's bothering you and approximately how long they require. Ask for some guidelines. Make sure he possesses guidelines. No, he cannot rationally say, "You have such and such a neurosis that I think can be treated effectively in twenty-six one-session weeks." But he *can* indicate the length of time similar cases have taken and, above all, from this can evolve a plan for the therapy.

The way he responds will give you an idea of what he *really* thinks—whether he'd *like* the therapy to last only several months, for example, but may be subliminally telling you that several years are going to be necessary. In turn, you must know what your own feelings are about the different lengths of time the therapy can consume. If you are going into therapy for the right reason, if you truly have a focal problem you earnestly want to resolve, you will also intuitively know fairly accurately how long that should require. Tune into your time frame. Discover it.

Still, important as it is to discuss the ending at the beginning, termination cannot be scheduled. What *can* be done, though, is to set up points along the way to check and recheck your progress, to see whether you are closer to termination than the last week, and the week before. Therapy can easily become narcotic. The means can subtly, malignantly replace the end.

One of the best thinkers on therapy is Dr. Richard D. Chessick, associate professor of psychiatry at Northwestern University. His book *Why Psychotherapists Fail* is dedicated "to my patients, especially those who have experienced with me the tragedy of failure in psychotherapy," and he has the honesty to speak of one of his own cases where "the most remarkable fact about this therapy, which lasted about two hundred hours, was that absolutely nothing happened at all! The patient continued unchanged in every way for two years. . . ." If this can occur with such a sensitive psychotherapist as Chessick, it seems next to impossible that therapy could ever be successful with a shrink to whom it is *un*remarkable that many hours pass without progress. One of the most successful therapists I talked to was Dr. Billy Sharp, a psychologist who is able to help people not only with their "inner" conflicts but rapidly and permanently with "visceral" life problems such as smoking, overweight, alcoholism, and job and marital conflicts. His views on termination are firm and fervent in the following interview:

So few therapists I have talked to have even thought about termination. But it seems to me that unless the therapist has given a lot of thought and talked about termination right from the outset with the patient, the therapy between them almost has to come to no good. What do you do about termination?

People become dependent, and you have to be very careful not to have that become a long-term state. When they do become too dependent, for too long, or they no longer need therapy, I think termination is necessary.

Generally, I handle it by scheduling appointments at greater intervals. I'll say to them, "I think what we ought to do now is take what we've talked about and what you've learned and use it for a month. Then give me a call and we'll schedule an appointment to come back." The next time I'll spread it out to two months or something like that. *I deliberately terminate people.*

How do you approach the subject?

I used to start out and ask people what their goals were, what they wanted out of psychotherapy, but I discovered that this approach didn't work too well. So now I start out with *problems.* Once we've solved a couple of problems, I'll introduce the subject of termination. "What do you want out of this now? . . . I just want to be sure why you came to see me in the first place . . . What were the problems you were dealing with? . . . Now that we've looked at some of those, what do you want you of this relationship?" These are some of the questions I ask them fairly soon. In that way, goals for the therapy—and particularly the terminating of the therapy—are established. It won't work to ask people what their goals were at the outset, because they actually don't know until they've worked with a couple of problems. But once they see they can solve problems, that seems to break the barrier. Then they can talk with me about what they've learned, and see that they can handle other problems by themselves.

What would be the main criticism by other therapists, right or wrong, of your method?

If anyone would criticize my approach in this regard, the criticism would probably be that I terminate people too quickly. They might say that I leave people before they have all their problems solved and all their goals reached. My approach is a little unusual. I rarely see anyone for a year. What I often do is see people for eight or ten sessions. Then they go away and stay away for a period of time, call me back and tell me they'd like to come in for a couple more sessions. Something else had happened in their lives, and they didn't quite know how to apply what we had worked on in therapy. It happened just this morning. A woman called and said she knew exactly what she wanted to do, and scheduled three sessions. I may never see her again after those three, because she'll learn more concepts she can apply. Or she may come back for some later problem in her life years from now.

Focusing on the positive and moving to it quickly is like planting a tree and nurturing it properly. An occasional weed nearby isn't that significant. And if the weed does get big enough, we can always tackle it with a few more sessions.

But your method doesn't work with everybody, does it?

Oh, of course there are people it doesn't work with. I have a telephone number written down in front of me right now, for instance, of a young woman I'm going to call and see how things are going, because I terminated her about six to eight weeks ago, and she wasn't very comfortable with the termination. Yet, I may find out that things are going well for her.

What about the other end of the spectrum—psychoanalysis?

Extensive psychoanalysis? At one point in my life I felt it was worthwhile. But now it has the potential to create a terribly dependent relationship. Anything like six or eight or ten years would make me feel there was something wrong. The process shouldn't take that long. I would say that this might be buying friendship, and I much prefer to encourage someone to find friendship—or related things that could be better found elsewhere than in a therapist's office.

Would you vary your approach if someone were hospitalized with a breakdown?

I might spend a little more time in the initial phases of problem-solving, but my approach would be pretty much the same. You see, some people don't want to solve their problems. All they want is friendship, or that listening ear. I happen to think that isn't beneficial if it continues too long.

I was trained in the psychoanalytic theory of therapy, the purpose of which is true regression, to take you back to the dependent relationship of your early years and get the transference going, ultimately bringing you up to the point where you and the therapist would be friends. I guess you could say that such an approach is for a small percentage of people who need help. I went through classical psychoanalysis, and I think part of it was beneficial to me. But the analyst was not at all willing to terminate me when I terminated. She thought I was making a very serious mistake in terminating at that time. I don't feel I made a mistake.

But you were trained to become a therapist. The average person wouldn't have that training, and might not be able to have the autonomy within the situation to terminate or the knowledge of how to go about it, true?

True, I was trained by a couple of people who were analyzed by Freud himself, and I think they felt that it had worked for them. But I don't think analysis is for most people. And in my practice I always feel it's up to *me* to put termination in focus and make it an issue. The therapeutic goal, you know, is for a person to take control of his or her own life, not to have somebody else take control of it. You could say that the overall goal of therapy is that the therapist should as soon as possible, and no longer, be necessary to the patient.

In *The Denial of Death* Ernest Becker says: "In this sense, as Rank saw with such deep understanding, psychoanalysis actually stultifies the emotional life of the patient. Man wants to focus his love on an absolute measure of power and value, and the analyst tells him that all is reducible to his early conditioning and is therefore relative. Man wants to find and experience the marvelous, and the analyst tells him how matter-of-fact everything is, how clinically explainable are our deepest ontological motives and guilts. Man is thereby deprived of the absolute mystery he needs, and the only omnipotent thing that then remains is the man who explained it away. And so the patient clings to the analyst with all his might and dreads terminating the analysis."

What is true of psychoanalysis is also true to a lesser degree of every kind of formal therapy. Termination of psychotherapy, like crossing a chasm with a couple of pretty good leaps and one small leap, is not one of those things that can be done *almost* right.

10
How to Find, Interview, and Save Money on the Right Therapist

We spend a huge amount of time and dollars checking out everything from the autos we drive to the markets where we shop and spend almost no time at all checking out the mind that does all that checking. If we become physically ill, we will pay through the nose for five minutes with a doctor and for the pills he prescribes. But what about our mental health?

Mental health is worth money. A recent University of Illinois study showed that people working at substantially less than emotional or mental well-being make approximately 40 percent less income than they could otherwise earn. Little problems, like "little" illnesses, don't always go away by themselves. If you fail to attend to them while they are still small, they can cost you a lot of money. On the other hand, therapy can be the biggest of financial ripoffs.

For one thing, therapy is generally too expensive. Most of those nearly twenty million Americans who spent more than twenty billion dollars last year on their mental health could not afford it. Second, they usually don't get what they are paying for. There is a way to save a great deal of money and still have good psychotherapy. But first you must ascertain whether you really need therapy. Ask yourself these questions:

1. Do I have some specific, long-standing habit or problem that, more than being simply a problem in itself, is affecting other areas of my life?
2. Am I frequently depressed or subject to attacks of anxiety without knowing the reason for them?
3. Do I lack people in my life with whom I can talk out my problems?

A "yes" answer to more than one of these questions is an indication that you might profit from therapy. And remember that you need not have deep-seated or complicated neuroses in order to want help. Samuel W. had the problem of shyness, a much commoner problem than most people might imagine. It held him back from being promoted in his job, as well as inhibiting his social life. At the age of forty he seemed to be getting worse rather than better (which is still another crucial measure of whether you should see a therapist).

After a dozen visits to a psychologist much of Samuel's fear was allayed. He began speaking before small groups. The more he did so, the more the fear vanished, until, a year later, his company noticed the change and expanded his duties. Soon after, he was promoted and now earns $12,000 more annually than he did a few years ago.

Other common problems for which short-term psychotherapy can sometimes be of help are:

—Hostility between parents and children
—Problem drinking
—Overweight
—Heavy smoking
—Phobias

The kinds of problems that stand a much smaller chance of success with even a very good therapist are:

—Sexual problems (especially homosexuality)
—Alcoholism
—-Criminal tendencies
—Basic personality traits (such as moodiness or a cynical outlook)
—Financial pressures

Regarding the problem area of financial worries, an important fact to keep in mind is this: Not only is therapy generally unable to improve our financial situation, or any other, but psychotherapy itself often becomes an additional financial burden.

All the more reason to find the right therapist.

Ann Landers, in her column of October 13, 1980, asserts that "a personal recommendation from a satisfied patient is the best referral." *Personal* is the crucial word here, because "reputation" means little in the field of psychotherapy. A man may be well known because he has had articles or books published. This does not necessarily make him a good therapist.

Still, a referral is only the beginning of your search. Unless the referral is from someone pretty much in a life situation similar to yours, it may not be worth while. It's also important to know the kind of shrink recommended. Broadly, these are the main categories, though it should be noted that they overlap greatly:

Psychoanalyst   A medical doctor who is licensed by the state after completing medical school, internship, and several years of residency. Most psychoanalysts believe in long-term therapy, going back to the patient's childhood at great length and in great detail to locate what they believe to be the source of the individual's present problems. A number of psychoanalysts, however, have abandoned this method for more conventional and shorter-term psychotherapy.

68

Psychiatrist	The same qualifications as a psychoanalyst, but with no commitment to long-term analysis or extensive investigation into early life as a method of treatment.
Psychologist	Not a medical doctor, but, in most states, a degree from a postgraduate program approved by the American Psychological Association is required. Usually, an internship with an agency dealing in mental health and passing an exam for this specialty is also needed.
Psychiatric Social Worker	None of the above qualifications, but specialized training, usually in personal counseling. A master's degree in social work is also necessary.
Psychiatric Nurse	A registered nurse who has been trained to some extent in psychotherapy. She has not, however, passed any specialized exam, nor is she registered by the state as more than a nurse.
Counselor	A person who may have *no* specialized training at all, nor any certification to practice psychotherapy. However, as long as such an individual does not pur-

port to have credentials he doesn't possess, he is generally allowed by law to counsel people just as a psychiatrist or psychologist might.

Once you have found a psychotherapist you feel may be right for you, the only way to make sure is to spend a session with him. Some psychologists will be willing to talk with you for twenty minutes or so, at no charge. Usually, however, especially with therapists who have a medical degree, you will have to pay for the "interview."

It may seem strange that *you* should interview the *therapist,* but it is important for these reasons: (1) It will give you a feeling of whether the two of you can get along (and no relationship will work, particularly therapy, unless the two people are in "synch" as human beings). (2) It sets up, at the outset, your autonomy in the relationship. Too often, patients simply abdicate their own independent roles in therapy from the beginning, and soon become extremely dependent upon the therapist. Whatever help they gain while going to the therapist vanishes when they attempt to leave therapy.

Pertinent questions to ask a therapist are these:

"Why do you think you can help me?"
"Why did you become a therapist?"
"Have you seen people with problems similar to mine?"
"How long do you feel I will need to be in therapy?"

Inappropriate questions are:

"What do you think of me?"
(How can a therapist possibly know? Besides, you aren't there for his approval; you're there for his help.)
"Can you cure me?"
(A complete "cure" of *any* problem is unlikely, and can be done only by the patient after "successful" therapy.)
"Will treating this problem make some of my other problems go away?"
(Treating one's major problems usually does help in other areas, but there is no guarantee.)

Interviewing at least several different therapists before deciding is a good investment. You may have to resist the temptation to go back to the first therapist you saw, primarily because he *was* the first. You may, in fact, decide *not* to go into therapy at all after two or three such interviews. For even if you are well off financially, therapy can be a drain, and the drain can be an irritation. That irritation can mask other problems, or create them. Few of us are sufficiently well-off in this inflationary economy to afford three sessions of psychoanalysis a week at $75 per session. In a feature story on "The Psychic Cost of Inflation" *Time* quoted Dr. Alan Grouber, a Massachusetts psychologist, as saying: "The people we see would ordinarily be able to cope, but with inflation they can't cope now. It is just too much."

What they have to cope with, *Time* further reported, was this: "Fees for a therapy session vary widely, roughly from $15 to $100 an hour, depending on the locality and reputation of the therapist. In Manhattan the average session cost $45 to $50 three years ago, $60 to $75 today." In the year and a half since that survey was taken, prices have gone considerably higher.

You may be able, however, to cut psychotherapy costs in the following ways:

1. *Remember that money spent on therapy is a medical tax deduction.*   Naturally, your tax bracket is instrumental in how much of a saving can exist.

2. *Attempt to have the psychotherapist lower the fee.* Many therapists will indeed do this, but not unless *you* bring up the subject. As *Time* said: "For years psychiatrists have been regarded as medicine's robber barons. But in fact, as medical specialists go, they rank relatively low on the pay scale." No one will ever hold a benefit for psychiatrists. But, unlike physicians per se—or lawyers or electricians—the prime motive of many therapists is genuinely to help people. As long as they make a good living doing it, they will occasionally adjust their fees if someone truly needs help.

3. *Shop around.* Just as with any other item you buy as a consumer, you will usually go wrong by taking the first price you are given. Psychotherapy is a field where the people who charge the highest prices are not necessarily the most competent. The more dedicated therapist wants mainly to make a good living and does not gouge.

4. Finally, *know how to end therapy.* "Termination" —the rational, mutual ending of therapy between patient and therapist—is something the patient must initiate. You must go into therapy with a certain time/money limit in mind, and stay within that framework. You should not linger on unless you absolutely must. It is better to leave the therapist temporarily and go back. Only by leaving him can you discover if the "help" you've been given can be turned into *self*-help.

11
After Therapy

Even successful termination is sometimes a bittersweet experience. As with everything of value in life, something must be given up—time if nothing else—for something greater to be gained. A successfully terminated psychotherapeutic relationship is rare; naturally, the patient—and the therapist—feel some loss. But the therapist has other patients; the patient has no other therapist. How do you deal with this?

First, know that you don't have to deal with it. To leave *professional* therapy if that therapy was successful, is to be able then to *gain* therapy from others who are nonprofessionals, yet who can now help more. As has been noted before, long before there were psychiatrists and psychologists, there was *psychotherapy.* It came from religious leaders, from our families, friends, neighbors, from books, and even, simplistic as it sounds, from a sunny day.

After Therapy

For me, because the written word is so important in my life, half a dozen passages in various pieces of literature can alter my mood significantly for the better, sometimes even seem to solve my problems. One is the poem "Excelsior!" by Longfellow:

The shades of night were falling fast. . . .
As through an Alpine village passed. . . .
A youth, who bore 'mid snow and ice,
A banner with a strange device,
    Excelsior!
His brow was sad, his eye beneath
Flashed like a falchion
    from its sheath. . . .
And like a silver clarion rung
The accents of that unknown tongue,
    Excelsior!
In happy homes he saw the light
Of household fires gleam
    warm and bright. . . .
Above, the spectral glaciers shone,
And from his lips escaped a groan,
    Excelsior!
'Try not the pass,'
    the old man said. . . .
'Dark lowers the tempest overhead,
The roaring torrent is deep and wide!'
And loud that clarion voice replied,

Excelsior!
'Oh, stay,' the maiden said, 'and rest
Thy weary head upon this breast!'
A tear stood in his bright blue eye. . . .
But still he answered with a sigh,
    Excelsior!
'Beware the pine tree's
    withered branch!'
'Beware the awful avalanche!'
This was the peasant's last good-night,
A voice replied far up the height,
    Excelsior!
At break of day as heavenward
The pious monks of St. Bernard
Uttered the oft-repeated prayer. . . .
A voice cried through the startled air,
    Excelsior!
A traveller, by the faithful hound,
Half-buried in the snow was found. . . .
Still grasping in his hand of ice
That banner with its strange device,
    Excelsior!
There in the twilight cold and gray,
Lifeless, but beautiful, he lay. . . .
And from the sky serene and far,
A voice fell, like a falling star,
    'Excelsior!'

Why the entire poem? Not as a panacea—each of us responds differently to different stimuli. But because merely *naming* something without *knowing* it is to imitate one of psychotherapy's common mistakes. However, I have given the poem to a number of people who were depressed, and it seemed to provide most of them with some insight or sense of life that removed their depression, at least temporarily. Once I was arguing the merits of "Excelsior!" with Robert Cosbey, then professor of English at Roosevelt University and one of the two finest teachers *I* ever encountered. He contended that "Excelsior!" was not a great poem because, unlike "Paradise Lost," more was not gained from each successive reading.

"But can't you gain something each time," I asked, "not for the mind, but for the soul? And must you see something new? Can't it be a renewal of something valuable that you've known before?"

Professor Cosbey was silent for a moment. I asked him what he was thinking. "I was remembering the last time I criticized "Excelsior!" to a class," he smiled. "Afterward a man about thirty came up to me and said he wanted me to know that once when he'd been seriously considering suicide, that poem had turned him away from it."

For some of us poems don't mean a thing. It might be an exciting sporting event or hearing an uplifting piece of music. Or, oftener, one or a few special people in our lives. Virtually any relationship is in some part psychotherapy.

A second accomplishment of successful termination is to build those bridges with others *during* therapy. Then, when we leave, we go to what we need, and our need to go back is less. One former patient who went to a therapist for the better part of a year, and smoothly, mutually terminated with her therapist, told me: "Most of my friends who went to therapists are still seeing them, or seeing another therapist. Half a dozen different psychiatrists and one psychologist are involved. They don't seem to want their patients to leave. But I found a man who brought up how long the whole thing should take right from the beginning. Before that, I went a few times to someone else, but I could see that he was someone who wanted to go on for as long as possible. He was bright, and I gained a good deal of insight from the three sessions I had with him, but the insights didn't really have any effect on my life. I brought up leaving within a few more weeks if I didn't get reasonably better quickly, and I could tell he was shocked and angry. I stopped going to him immediately and found a better therapist. I still remember ten minutes into that very first meeting, when I was about to ask him about how long he thought it would take, he brought up the subject. He said once a week, anywhere from six to eight months. That's exactly how long it did take."

She went on: "An aspect of what was giving me difficulty came down to problems with my husband and one child in particular. The therapist helped me to improve my relationships with them, to the point where my husband now actually is a therapist for me and I for him. And I think I'm a pretty good therapist for my child when she needs it. I've gravitated more toward a couple of friends with whom I can receive and give help in that way when we need it, and I'm seeing some of the old friends less. It might seem strange, but there are also a couple of television programs that are of enormous help when I'm in a state of anxiety. 'Mr. Rogers' is one of them. Just listening to him, hearing his therapeutic approach, invariably puts me back on the right track. I don't think I'll ever see a professional therapist again."

The point is that if termination is successful, the patient, truly helped by therapy, will *already have* the tools for self-therapy *before* the sessions end. For the patient whose therapy has been unsuccessful and whose termination was not a segue but a rupture, there will be a mushrooming need to return the same time, next week.

12
In Bed–and in Love
–with the Therapist

The twenty-six-year-old woman is intelligent, well proportioned, with a pretty face and a fetching, outgoing personality. But she is a troubled woman, having recently broken up with a lover after an affair that lasted three years. Before that, she was married briefly and divorced. She is highly sexual, has chosen men for her partners who are highly sexual, yet cannot seem to sustain a relationship with the opposite sex after a few months. A few months ago she was sitting in a psychiatrist's office, her fifteenth visit, and was finally about to reveal her sexual fantasies.

"I guess what I want most," she confided, "is to be tied up. If I were tied, and I completely trusted the man, I could let him do the things to me which really turn me on. I'm not just talking about oral intercourse, which obviously I've done and enjoy. But I know I'd enjoy it more, really be turned on, if I were tied up and I *couldn't* resist it. I just haven't been able to trust any man that much. Once I let Ted, whom I have just broken up with, tie my wrists behind me to the headboard, but my legs were free, and I ended up kicking him in the face when he was going to do exactly one of the things I wanted him to do!"

The young woman went on in greater detail and, as she did, noticed more than the usual interest on the part of her therapist. He began asking her other questions regarding her sexual preferences. As she left the office that day, he touched her for the first time, an affectionate squeeze on the shoulder. It both bothered her and stirred her up. Did he mean more by it than merely a gesture of support?

She found out soon after. The therapist asked her out socially, and within a month, they were sleeping together, he catering to her exact sexual fantasies. He is married, and has four children. Currently, she still sees him as a therapist, but often with the door to his office locked.

A fifty-four-year-old man reveals an essentially similar experience:

"Natalie and I had what I thought was a good marriage. It was the second for each of us, and we felt we'd really done it right this time around. We did have problems, the main one being a lack of sexual interest on her part most of the time. But we'd weathered many larger problems. And, so help me, we were in love. I didn't think there was anything that could shake our marriage.

"Two years ago, Natalie suggested we each go into therapy separately to try and make things more romantic in bed. I chose a psychologist a few years older than myself, a man, and Natalie decided to see a female psychiatrist. For the first few months it seemed to help both of us. We discussed what was going on with our therapists, and the exchange, if nothing else, seemed good. But then Natalie became guarded when it came to talking about her sessions. She increased to twice a week, and seemed to draw further from me rather than closer. A period began, which was never to end, where we had no sex at all. She said that until she worked out her problems, she didn't want to take a chance on compounding them. I didn't like that, but decided to abide by it for a while.

"Almost a year to the day Natalie began her therapy she told me one night that she had thought things over and wanted a divorce. It hit me like a ton of bricks. Our children were grown, and we'd always both talked about spending the rest of our lives together once the kids were gone, doing just what we liked to do together. I'd done well financially from the time I was in my middle forties, so we could afford to. Anyway, after I got myself together, I tried to fight it. 'Look—we went to solve our problems,' I told her. 'What can you have found out that would make you want a divorce after we've gone through so much together and stayed together?'

"The worst thing was that she refused to discuss it. She said that was what she wanted, and she had a right to live apart from me as she chose. I could argue that, but I was shattered. I pleaded with her for a trial separation, with both of us keeping up our therapy and possibly getting back together. But she wanted a divorce flat out. I gave it to her.

"From that point on Natalie wanted very little contact with me. Two months later I found out from a third party that she had given up her own apartment and moved in with her therapist. They were having an affair. Since then, even though it's been only a relatively short time, she's left her therapist and gone to two other females. I've talked to enough people to know that though we did have our problems sexually, our relationship in that way wasn't much different from that of most married couples. And I had been close to Natalie long enough to *know* she really isn't a lesbian. I think she just got involved with this therapist, who obviously was a confirmed homosexual, and was persuaded to throw everything over for her.

"I still can't believe it happened. I can't believe it would have happened, either, if Natalie hadn't gone to this therapist. She still sees the woman, though they don't live together. For a long time I felt there was something wrong with *me* because of it. But now I've talked to enough people to realize that it isn't uncommon for lives to be changed by what the therapist says or does, and that a lot of therapists become personal with their patients."

These two cases, though they might seem somewhat bizarre, are not rare exceptions. Not long ago *Newsweek,* in reporting the case of a New Jersey woman suing her psychiatrist for $450,000 because he had supposedly ruined her marriage and her mental health by seducing her, cited a further survey indicating that as high as 8 percent of all therapists are involved in sexual relationships with their patients. The true figure may be higher, because most patients would not want such a relationship publicized and virtually no therapist does, since a sexual liaison with a patient could be grounds for malpractice.

Recently, even "Dear Abby" printed a letter from a woman who had been married seventeen years and who had fallen hopelessly in love with her therapist. In 1979, *Psychology Today* reported the findings of a study by the American Psychological Association, where it was found that many female psychotherapists had begun sexual contact with their own teachers as far back as graduate school. The study saw the figure going higher. Less than 2 percent of the therapists interviewed felt that sexual contact with clients could ever be healthful. Yet obviously a significant number of therapists indulge in sexual relations with their clients, whether or not it is good for the patient.

Sexual relations with the therapist do not *have* to take place, however, in order for there to be sexual problems between patient and therapist. Sexual *feelings* toward the therapist, especially women toward a male therapist, are overwhelmingly common. In fact, the first dictum of psychoanalysis is "transference," where crucial feelings,

84

some of which are inevitably sexual, are put onto the therapist before the psychotherapeutic process can work. Though most therapy today is not psychoanalytic in the strict sense, a mini-transference often occurs. If the therapist is not an object of at least some attraction, in fact, the patient's motivation may be less. Who would want a therapist who does not seem strong and capable? And it is our early perception of the desirability and capability, or lack of them, of the parent of the opposite sex that usually has the most influence upon our sexual feelings. Our sexuality is diffuse when we are three, six, or even ten, yet powerful. A little girl may not explicitly fantasize intercourse with her father, or a boy with his mother, but *that* is the subconscious psychic prize of winning the affection of that parent. Those unidentified and unresolved childhood feelings, brought forth in any therapeutic process, now devolve on the therapist, explicitly.

If this were not the case, most women would not go to male therapists, and so many men to female psychologists and psychiatrists (and there is evidence that more men would go to female therapists if the preponderance of males in the field were not so heavy).

Ordinarily, we can handle sexual attraction toward someone else. But when it is our therapist, it is a different matter. And what if the therapist *cannot* handle the patient's sexual feelings toward him?

If sex with one's psychotherapist is destructive, it is at least blatantly destructive. Much more common, and much more insidious, is *love*, of one type of another, for one's therapist.

A thirty-six-year-old man reveals this not untypical situation:

"I began seeing T—— three years ago. I had a good marriage, two nice kids, an expensive condominium, money in the bank, and was on the way up in my career —had everything, as I look back on it. But I was depressed —nothing world-shaking, just off-and-on depression. But it disturbed me, and it disturbed my wife, because I had always been the kind of person who hardly ever got depressed. I had what was commonly called a very positive mental attitude toward life. I almost liked obstacles so that I could have the thrill of overcoming them. Nothing stopped me.

"How many times I've wished that I could go back to that time, that I had fought my way through those mild depressions as I did everything else. Instead, I went to see a psychologist. She was nearby, so it was convenient, and I only intended to go for a few weeks. If you had told me at the beginning that I'd end up falling in love with T— I would have said you were crazy. I remember clearly seeing her for the first time. Physically, she was everything my wife wasn't—and I find my wife *very* attractive. My wife is tall, slender, very graceful and beautiful, and you can't mistake the fact that she is a female. T—— was much shorter, certainly not attractive by my standards or those of most people, and she was older than I am. And my mother didn't look like that either, by the way. In fact, one of the reasons I felt secure seeing her—I'd never committed adultery in my marriage—was because I knew I would not be attracted to her as a woman and would not have to worry about that. She's not overweight, but is kind of a thick-bodied person, and I had never been attracted to that type of woman. One of the things I've learned through therapy is that our physical preferences are based on deeper psychological feelings. Nevertheless, my inner feelings certainly had never made a woman like that seem attractive in the past.

"She *did* help me in the beginning. But the price I paid for it is far greater than any help I received. She helped me to see that the depression I had been going through off and on was only veiled anger. Against what? Against exactly the kind of nice, stable life I'd been leading. Yes, I had everything, so to speak, but those of us who pursue something very strongly and live rather rigidly within it are always candidates, I guess, for the very opposite. I'd known about ambivalent feelings before I went into therapy, but another thing that T—— showed me, and rather quickly, was how each thing can generate its own opposite in many people. I could tell you so many things I've learned through her, but I'd feel like the man who has gained the world and lost himself. I have all this knowledge about myself, but now I'm hopelessly in love with T——, can't leave her, and every other part of my life has suffered because of this.

"It had nothing to do with transference. Well, It does, but not in the classic psychoanalytic sense. T—— doesn't believe in any of that nonsense. But it can happen anyway, and I know a classic Freudian analyst would say that I'm only going through it and some day will come out of it. Well, I've been waiting for that some day for the last year and a half and I don't see it ever happening. I'm in love with her, helplessly so, and who's to say what love is? My feeling toward my wife hasn't changed that much. Now, though, it's not as important a feeling as what I have for T——.

"Because she did help me in the beginning, I decided to go for a few months instead of a few weeks. I guess that was my first mistake, except that one thing always leads to another if the elements are there, and the real mistake was going at all. After four and a half months, I did decide to leave, nevertheless. I remember walking out of her office on that last day that wasn't the last day. It was raining out, but I felt good. My depression had been pretty much relieved, and was becoming milder all the time, and I was going back to the life I was satisifed with, even though part of me at times wanted to throw it all over, just chuck the responsibilities and go traveling around the world. Now that I understood that this had been what was bothering me and giving me this repressed anger I was covering up and turning into depression, I wasn't as depressed and the need to get away from it all wasn't as pressing. I was elated that I had gone for a problem and overcome it. Seeing a therapist was simply a new way to overcome it, just as you might go to a gas station down the road to get your tire fixed. Or at least that's the way I prefer to think of it.

"That night at dinner I still felt in excellent spirits. My wife and I related beautifully, and later on we went to bed and made love for the first time in weeks. And it was good, very good. I was slightly disturbed that once or twice during the lovemaking itself I though of T——. She just popped into my head. It bothered me not to be totally involved in the lovemaking every second. Still, as I said, it was very good. That night I had trouble getting to sleep, and when I did, I dreamed about the lovemaking, but it was T——'s face on my wife's body. I had the same dream a few nights later. And when we tried to make love, for the first time in my life I couldn't get an erection. I had always been intensely attracted to my wife, and this really disturbed me. It sent me back to T——.

"It disturbed me to go back, because it introduced the question of whether I had ever really been through with therapy in the first place. Now I could not say I was going only for a few sessions. I felt as if I had lost some control of the therapeutic situation, and it's important for me to have reasonable control over anything I do. But when I walked out of T——'s office after that first return session, I realized for the first time that I wasn't back for any problem. I was back for T——.

"I can't tell you the exact point at which I knew I was

in love with her. I realize how horribly trite this seems, for I'm in a medically related job and have heard many women tell how they fell in love with their male therapist. I used to have to fight not to laugh when someone said that. But it happens. If it can happen to me, it can happen to anyone. My guess is that it happens quite often, and I don't know how you get out of it. I'm still going to T——, and I think she knows what I feel, although we don't discuss it explicitly in the sessions, but deal with it in a more roundabout way. I do not believe she truly loves me. But she does have a certain kind of respect for me, and I sense she is attracted to me, and so there is a basis for a relationship, even though the relationship can't go outside the office. Sometime, though, I may tell her exactly what I feel. I don't know. I'm so confused. It seems absolutely insane to think of divorcing your wife for your therapist, especially when there's not a chance in a thousand that the therapist is interested that way in you. And I don't really think about divorcing my wife. I wouldn't want to do that, wouldn't want to marry T—— if somehow it could all be worked out. I like my life the way it is. But because I've fallen in love with T——, my life isn't what it was. My marital relationship is having more and more difficulty, which I talk about with T——. I wouldn't say my work is suffering, but it isn't moving forward as it should. I don't care as much about working out and keeping in shape as I used to. Everything is up and down. But what isn't up and down is this relationship I've gotten myself into and can't get myself out of. I don't even think of leaving therapy any more. I only hope that nothing changes so that I can keep going to see her a couple of times a week. That's why I haven't told her exactly what I feel. I'm afraid she might want to cut the therapy short, though she hasn't given any indication of that. It's a mess, a ruddy mess. What I wouldn't give to go back to the days of off-and-on simple depressions. No, I wasn't facing them squarely, but who needed it? I really didn't have that much to be depressed about. Now I do."

Clearly it is difficult to keep personal involvement *out* of the picture while the therapist and patient are still involved *enough* to get the work done. Thus, in still another manner psychotherapy can be a cure worse than the illnesses it purports to treat.

13
Psychotherapy in a Capsule

There is a great deal of evidence, most of it still controversial, that drug therapy, not unlike life-support machines, (1) can keep alive the terminally psychotic, (2) can render somewhat functional—at what ultimate cost is not known —the essentially nonfunctioning neurotic, and (3) temporarily stabilize the patient undergoing a breakdown in preparation for therapy.

But only pill-less therapy can take it from there, and take it to where it must lead. Yes, the mind is made of of physical cells, and the implication is that those cells are treatable by certain chemcials, just as the body is. The grave questions the brave new world of therapeutic pharmacology raises are these:

—Are most drugs we take for even nonpsychological, strictly physical ills doing us more harm than good in the long run?

Psychotherapy in a Capsule

—If therapy does not understand the human mind
 enough to treat it successfully without drugs, how can
 it presume to treat the human psyche with them?
—Is the prescribing of pills by a psychiatrist inherently
 destructive to his relationship with the patient?

I interviewed a man who had been in and out of
therapy for ten years. His neuroses were fairly severe and,
though the therapy had not helped him, he had always
been able to stay on the right side of the edge, had a good
marriage and a flourishing career. In his mid-fifties, after
three years without therapy, he went to a psychiatrist who
prescribed drugs for his condition.

The condition improved. But the patient didn't.

The man's neuroses bothered him less now, but he
gradually lost some of his ambition. He gained weight, his
marriage suffered, and, eventually, his physical health.
Finally, he left the therapist, went off the pills and didn't
return to either pills or therapy. His physical condition
improved, his ambition returned. And his severe neuroses
did too. He'd just have to live with them, he decided, but
at least he would be living fully as what he is.

The man left therapy because it had failed him. The
therapist's pills, however, had "succeeded," though not in
giving him relief from his neuroses *while still allowing
him to retain what was most important to him in life.*

Thus, going to a series of therapists, culminating in the pill-prescriber, had made him see that professional therapy could not help him. Actually, the pills had done exactly what he had wanted his therapists to do. In reality, the pills were only an extension in chemical form of the therapeutic methodology and thus of the therapist himself. But because of their immediacy, their elimination of the therapist's fallacies and of the patient's digressions, and because they could be taken every day and every night, they had worked.

In seeing this, what the patient saw was that the pills were not the answer for him and, most certainly, therapists were not, because they had been only a milder version of the tablets he had been swallowing. Too many patients have not learned, though, that the 50¢ capsule chemical cannot basically succeed when a $50-an-hour aspirin has failed. It is no accident that the current therapeutic craze of our culture, Valium, has the adverse side effect of lowering the white cell count in a number of people after extended use. The while cells are, of course, those that fight illness.

Except in psychotic or emergency situations, pills are a very dubious way of treating emotional and mental illness. Whether they work or not, drugs profoundly denigrate the efficacy of therapy. The therapist who prescribes them is really acting as a physician. Well, 75 million American prescribe their own drugs, mainly alcohol and/or marijuana. The growing use of both alcohol and marijuana is one of the many signals of a ground-level disenchantment with therapy. The issue of how harmful are alcohol and marijuana is not the minor issue. The major question is whether they are *less* harmful than the drugs psychiatrists would prescribe if these very same people went to them?

Psychologists prescribe drugs less than psychiatrists because their orientation is less medical, and because in most states they are not allowed to write prescriptions for drugs. Psychiatrists can do so easily. There are a group of medical therapists basically opposed to the use of drugs for the overwhelming majority of patients. They may not all be good therapists, but they have one asset the pill-prescribing psychiatrist does not possess: They have not relinquished their belief that psychotherapy can work.

A good question to ask a potential therapist when you interview him is what his views are on prescribing drugs within therapy. Those who are against it, except in special cases, are generally much better therapists. All things being equal, anyone who believes in what he is doing is better than someone who doesn't.

A therapist may tell you that a pill can be a substitute for will, but don't swallow it.

14
Therapy as Placebo

No matter how convincingly the case may be made for the glaring deficiencies today of therapy and most therapists, one imposing fact reoccurs: Some patients get better, with or without pills.

The important question is: *How many of these patients would have gotten better anyway?*

A placebo is a harmless and inactive "medicine" the doctor gives the unknowing patient in place of a real pill. My grandfather consistenly prescribed placebos for his patients with remarkable success, and was appalled by the extent to which other physicians overmedicated. If he were alive today, he would be even more shocked at the number of therapists who prescribe pills, and the kind of pills they prescribe. In many strictly medical conditions study after study has shown that placebos work as well as real medication. With patients who have emotional "illness" fewer studies have been made, but those that have been show the same results. What has *not* been examined and what seems abundantly true in many cases, is that *therapy itself* is the *placebo.*

Two and a half years ago a woman in her late fifties went to a therapist for the first time in her life. A year before she had lost her husband and was still depressed. Her daughter, who had gone into therapy because of marital problems—and divorced her husband seven months later—suggested that her mother see the same man. The woman did not go to the daughter's shrink. She was suspicious of him because the daughter's marital breakup was unnecessary in her judgment, and seemed to come about as a result of the therapy. But she did find another man and started seeing him. In a few sessions she felt well enough to leave. The therapist suggested she stay on, but she terminated anyway and is doing quite well. Her own feeling about why she was better after the therapy was this: "I believed it would help me, so it did help me. I don't think the psychologist did anything in particular to make me better. I just think I needed *something.*"

There are clearly many cases where therapy works, not because it really *works,* but because virtually *anything* would make the patient feel better. The patient is going to feel better anyway as long as he or she did do or take *something.* The *doing* by the *patient*, even the decision to do, is actually the cure.

One psychologist has told me: "I know most of my colleagues would publicly disagree with me, though a lot of them privately admit I'm right, but what I'm going to tell you is that I agree with Szasz that most people aren't emotionally ill but have only life problems. And most people who go to therapists aren't much different than those who don't. They're just more oriented toward therapy, usually. In my practice I've worked along a continuum, and done pretty well with it. And one aspect of the continuum, which is always where I begin, is that I look upon the therapy as a placebo. The patient simply wants to take something, as we often do for a headache. After one or two sessions, sometimes several more, the patient is better. My job is simply to be that something and to be nothing else, not to open up a can of worms.

"Next, if the placebo effect as a therapy doesn't do the job, I move a bit further down the continuum, to being a listener. It's remarkable how people will find their way and feel better if someone merely listens to them for an hour a week for awhile. After that a crucial point midway in my personal continuum of therapy is where there *is* a problem that needs working on, but where I don't look upon the patient as emotionally ill because of it. Then, of course, there is the other end of the continuum, where we have real illness, as we do in the body. That takes longer, but the patient has to prove to me that it should, that she or he is actually emotionally ill instead of just down or burdened by the weight of a temporary problem."

Not many therapists hold this view. To the extent that they don't—and to the extent that they intensively and extensively treat a person for illness rather than for living life—are they dangerous? Not for one minute do they allow therapy to be a placebo. Instead, they give strong medicine.

The patient was not sick. After this treatment, he is.

15
The $50-an-Hour Aspirin –
The Therapist as Anesthetist

Whether pills, placebo, or whatever, how often is the therapist ultimately merely an anesthetist?

Not long ago a man I know decided to visit his wife's psychiatrist for a single session to see if he could gain insight into improving certain aspects of his life.

"How are you?" the therapist began.

"Fine."

"Then why are you here?"

Twenty minutes later, after the man had been discussing what it was he felt could be improved, the therapist broke in. "But what *really* is your problem? You don't seem to be in pain."

The man had gone to the therapist for the rational reason of *avoiding future pain* as much as possible. But the therapist, like most psychiatrists and psychologists, was used to patients who had come only because their pain had become so severe that they had to seek out a therapist. If they had gone to a therapist, or done some hard thinking, *before* they were in great pain, then most of them would have avoided it. But we have become a no-pain-at-almost-any-cost culture, a society of cradle-to-grave soothing, a people who have forgotten the truth that pain is inextricably bound to joy. Is it a wonder, then, that we have become such a joyless population, constantly craving mere pleasure as a saccharine substitute. We expect and often demand automatic relief from the struggle of life, be it automatic raises that keep pace with inflation or the automatic raising of our spirits. And the apogee of this is the $50-an-hour aspirin administered by the psychotherapist.

A few years ago an intelligent, twenty-three-year-old single woman, the product of a divorced home with a rigid, guilt-giving father who drove another child into a mental institution, began seeing a therapist. Given her circumstances, she had made steady improvement and was developing a good life for herself, having attained a master's degree in sociology while holding down a $345-a-week position with a large market research firm. Today she is almost a basket case. She has not continued her education, as intended. Her job is in jeopardy from frequent absences. She is usually heavily sedated, under prescription of the psychiatrist, about whom her life revolves. She counts the days until her ten-thirty appointment each

Tuesday. If she has a "good" session, she feels better for a day or two. If the session does not relieve her pain, she plunges into an even deeper depression.

The therapist tells her she is "making progress." A fellow I knew once divorced his wife after six years of marriage, primarily, he said, because she had gained forty pounds and couldn't lose it. "Six years of marriage," he observed, "is enough time to lose forty pounds." Six years is enough time to make *tangible* progress. But not if one goes to a therapist mainly to allay present pain. And not if the therapist goes along. The relief from immediate pain can be a *by-product* of good therapy, but it cannot be therapy's *purpose*. To the extent it is, the patient will keep going and going, increasingly having to deal with the larger anguish of *only* relieving immediate pain. Eventually, the "fix" itself becomes a painful reproach, something desperately craved yet simultaneously saddening.

No one, except masochists, wants pain. Nor do we enjoy it when it comes our way. But the individual with a handle on autonomy and emotional health knows that certain kinds of pain are a necessary ingredient to his autonomy and health. Most of us, unfortunately, have become so "allergic" to virtually any kind of loss or failure that we retreat further and further into a corner of existence where our victories are less significant because we have less to lose.

The therapist who aids and abets us in this, whether out

of ignorant sympathy or a need for his own small successes, is no joy to behold.

Physically, pain is a valuable signal. It tells us something is wrong, but the *pain* itself is *not* what is wrong. With the exception of terminal diseases and short-term traumatic ruptures or fractures, pain is not nearly as painful as we have come to consider it. We overreact our pain, seldom differentiating one type of pain from another.

The same is true of psychological pain. It is no accident that euthanasia has become a leading issue in today's America, for here we have the ultimate relief of pain. Why is euthanasia such a fulminant issue? Mainly, it is because pain has become such an overwhelming issue for us. We have forgotten to value it, we hardly know how to deal with it, we have been led to believe we should never have to have it, and thus many of us can no longer even tolerate it to any degree. The mere thought of having pain endlessly evokes a frantic response from us.

Most psychotherapists, unthinkingly or deliberately, have been at the forefront of the no-pain parade. They are already administering euthanasia to the psyches of their willing patients.

16
The Therapist as Listener

Every Thursday after school, from November 1978 to
April 1979, Tim's mother would drive him to a leading
child psychologist. She would drop him off there shortly
before four, do some errands, pick him up at ten minutes
of five. From there, they'd drive home, dinner having
been prepared by the maid. Thirteen-year-old Tim went
to the psychologist at his mother's request, because he
hadn't been pulling grades as high as last year's, nor relating to his parents as well. Also, he had occasional temper
tantrums. Aside from this, he was pretty much like most
of his peers—in fact, these things may have made him
very much like most of his peers—but he did seem to
emerge from the sessions in a better mood. For one thing,
he was more civil at the dinner table. However, when his
parents would carefully ask him what he and the doctor

talked about, the boy's answers didn't seem to reveal any great truths of the universe to them. He talked pretty much about what most thirteen-year-old boys would talk about—his particular interests, not enough acceptance from his peers, conflicts with his parents, girls.

"Well, what did the doctor *say?*" they would probe.

"He doesn't say much of *anything*," Tim would shrug.

In early spring of 1979 Tim began to complain mildly that not only did the doctor not say much of anything, but that he didn't think he had much of anything to say to the doctor any more. It took him several weeks to convince his parents that he shouldn't go back. Finally, though, when the boy insisted, they gave in. "I wish he'd stayed longer," Tim's mother told her husband. "But I'm glad he went. I know it did him some good."

And indeed it did. The boy simply needed a listening ear.

Laura, a single woman of thirty-six, spends more than a third of her weekly paycheck as a teacher on twice-weekly visits to a therapist. Raised as a strict Catholic, she no longer follows her religion, but adheres to many of its moral scruples. This is one reason she had only one sexual encounter, which made her feel even more that she wanted no intimate relationship with a man unless it was intimate enough to result in marriage. She has never been close to her brother, and her parents retired to another part of the country. Highly intelligent, attractive, and hypersensitive to the possibility of being hurt in relationships, Laura has few friends, and, in fact, looks upon the therapist as her best friend. The one hundred minutes weekly she spends with him, though occasionally painfully introspective, are the most prized part of her week.

These two individuals are representative of many who go to therapists. Did the therapist make them feel better? Yes. But *because* he *wasn't* acting as a *therapist,* and *because* they were *not* there as *patients.*

One reason the therapist has become so popular in our culture is that he offers that all too rare commodity—*a listener.*

Our families, our friends, our coworkers *hear* us, but how often do they truly *listen?* The automobile that drove Tim to his weekly therapy session bore a bumper sticker on the back: HAVE YOU HUGGED YOUR KID TODAY? Tim's mother had hugged him every day. But had she listened to him?

We live in an information-geared society, and are so consumed by getting and spending information that in the process most of us lose the most human information. It begins early. Lecturing teachers of ever-larger classes seldom have time to hear anything but granite-hard facts or abstract theories bounced back to them, facts and theories leading to further facts and theories leading mostly to a place in that society where people earn their keep by punch-pressing out more facts and theories. This leaves only the child's parents, who usually are not good at parenting, and his peers, who are some solace, yet less and less, for they too have a crying need to be listened to. Finally, the ability to listen to ourselves is diminishing to the point of self-deafness. The continual thrum of our automobiles, the drone of our refrigerators and air conditioners, the cacophony of our TVs fill our ears. We no longer want to talk. We yearn to scream, and sometimes do.

Enter the therapist.

He listens. Is that bad?

It is often very bad. In a way, it is the ultimate "pill."

If the therapist is truly the *only* listener available, he will be providing an invaluable service. Where a man is not only widowed, but seen seldom by his children, and has no coworkers or neighborly neighbors, the fifty minutes weekly with a therapist could spell the difference between a depressive, even suicidal, state of mind and the maintenance of some happiness and will to live. It is hard to be old and alone in America.

However, much of what one is when one is older depends on what one was when younger. I have known a number of older men and women, suffering from severe, chronic physical problems, who found people to talk to. They keep working, if only as crossing guards or volunteers. They seek out companionship with the opposite sex through community and religious groups. They join health clubs, spending entire mornings, afternoons, or evenings there. They garden. They travel. And they meet people who are responsive and willing to listen, because *they* are so willing to listen, and the seeking out isn't that difficult, since there are so many older people in the same boat. Moreover, the relationships they find last longer than fifty minutes weekly and are more satisfying, for there is a mutuality of interest and situation.

The same goes for Laura and Tim. How many thirteen-year-olds have their grades fall when confronted by the new excitements and problems of puberty? And isn't this precisely the time when youngsters pull away from their parents and begin to move toward independence, frequently reestablishing the parent-child relationship later on an adult basis? If these are sufficient reasons to see a therapist, then almost every normal child in America should do so. The fact is that if his parents had cared less about his grades and more about truly listening to their son, they wouldn't have felt he needed a therapist to talk and listen to him.

With Laura, it may well be that her essentially solitary lifestyle was a matter of choice. There are quasi-hermits within as well as outside society. But then, isn't it a contradiction that she would feel the need, year after year, to be listened to by a therapist? At the very least doesn't it seem a waste for an intelligent, capable, fairly attractive thirty-six-year-old woman with no pressing emotional problems to have a therapist as her only friend?

Whatever the positive value may be to the person for whom a therapist is primarily a listener, there are inevitable and dangerous negatives.

First, displacement and dependence. Because the therapist is such an expert listener, other potential listeners seem to pale by comparison. It takes little effort to lie on a couch or sit in a chair for an hour and talk about ourselves to a captive audience. It usually requires a good deal more effort to pursue the give-and-take of talking to a nonpaid someone who is captivated by what we say only insofar as it is interesting, open, and balanced by our own ability to draw out and listen to what he or she has to say. With each additional fifty minutes the therapist knows more and more about us. That's a sure thing. And he "cares," because it's his job to care. Others in our life may really care much more, but how often do they give us uninterrupted moments of listening? So the patient who needs to be listened to begins to "save" what he or she has to say for that one audience that is certain to be attentive. The therapist inexorably displaces the potentially more rewarding but less predictable listeners; the patient becomes less dependent upon whether or not they listen, more dependent upon the therapist. The individual who enters the therapist's office because "I have no one to talk to, really" may unknowingly be embarking on a self-fulfilling prophecy.

Another danger of the therapist as listener is that he may do more than listen. He may open up the patient's own Pandora's box. All but the most zealous "let-everything-hang-out" shrink recognizes every person's need for adequate "defenses," which is something far different from being *defensive*. Therapy tends to weaken, sometimes demolish, our defenses. For those patients with a serious problem lurking behind the defense—or simply for those who for their own good reasons want to know "everything" about themselves—this is necessary. Handled like delicate brain surgery, it is beneficial. For the person with life's aggravating but average problems it can be highly detrimental.

Still another problem with the role of therapist as listener is that is is inherently demeaning to pay your listener. The man or woman who must pay a prostitute for sex—or who may prefer to—has a real problem. But wouldn't a person who pays someone to *listen* have even more of a problem? Which should be placed on a higher level, one's body or one's thoughts?

A man who buys sex, of course, is not merely demeaning his body. He is demeaning his mind. The act of paying someone to have sexual intercourse with him, whether it be a prostitute he buys for an hour or a partner he buys for several years by supporting her, implicitly says that he doesn't value himself enough to attempt to gain that intimacy based upon what he *is*.

Isn't the man or woman who pays for a special kind of social intercourse with a therapist saying much the same thing?

Yes, as that once popular song went, most of us just want someone we can talk to. That isn't the question. The question is should that someone be a therapist?

17
The Customer is Usually Wrong

Psychotherapy, *inherently*, has problems that may make it fail. Even when those problems are not a problem, the therapist may not be able to make psychotherapy succeed. But there *are* good therapists. Even so, all too often, it is the *patient* who insures that the therapeutic process will ultimately be a failure.

A damaging misconception that pervades our view of psychotherapy is that, if we can simply find a good therapist, more than half the battle is over. Far from it. The battle is over if we *don't* find a good therapist. But should we happen upon a competent and dedicated one, the chances against success weigh heavily against us, because of *ourselves*.

Mrs. H., for example, is *not* a vacuous, well-to-do woman who has very little to do. She is an intelligent, responsible mother of three with an avocation that earns her almost half of what her husband makes a year. Yet she spends the greater part of one day each week traveling to and from the suburbs for an appointment in a large city with a therapist. She has been doing this for almost two years now, and may do it for the rest of her life. Yet Mrs. H. doesn't go to the therapist because she is unusually neurotic, unhappy, or has any particular hangups that stultify her existence. She goes because it is part of her social life. Her friends go. Albeit, it is "the thing to do." Or at least, it's *something* to do.

Mrs. H. doesn't think of her "same time, next week" in those terms. Nor do the thousands of others who visit psychotherapists mainly to fill up their time or to fill in part of their social schedule. When one stops to think about it, it isn't a bad way to spend part of an afternoon. The therapist is usually supportive and seldom hostile, the "patient" can talk on and on if she wishes, and some small insight may even be gained through the process. It certainly beats going to the "right" supermarket to shop for groceries, and is more predictable than seeing the latest "in" movie on a weekend.

Have you ever overheard a couple of men or women talking endlessly about something of interest to them but essentially trivial to anyone else? A woman, for example, who gives a great many parties may spend forty-five minutes on the telephone with her friend talking about the arrangement of the seating. A man who spends his weekend watching football in front of the television may spend a majority of Monday talking about it to some buddy at the office. Well, they can do much the same with their therapist. No, they won't get the same feedback, but that will be more than compensated by the fact that they can usually go into great detail without interruption about why Mrs. Johnson should sit next to Mr. Arnold, or why the coach should have called a draw play on third and two.

This misuse of psychotherapy is widespread. Often the patient attempts to parlay the social hour at the therapist's office into socializing with the therapist outside the office. Many therapists allow this. The three principal reasons therapists allow themselves to be curried socially by their patients are: (a) fulfillment of their own neurotic needs, (b) social power, and (c) money. As to the first, one psychoanalyst explains; "Though it is probably wrong to do so, more and more psychiatrists and psychologists are throwing aside the accepted dictum that you do not socialize with your patients. I think that in large part this is happening because of the increased status of the therapist in our society and, simultaneously, an inadequate opportunity to *enjoy* that status. All day long the therapist must play the part—and a part it is—of more than a human being, of an objective standard. He learns the intimate details of people's lives, and may of course become emotionally involved with them. Yet virtually never can he really show his patients that he is human, and the need to do so burgeons with every passing month and year. Furthermore, therapists may not like to mingle with each other; they are weary of talking shop. This is precisely what they wish to escape from."

Nor is money to be ignored as a primary cause of the increasing tendency of therapists to socialize with their patients. As in any business, one contact leads to another. It pays to advertise, and the best advertisement is a good impression given in person. And, finally, the patient and —the patient's friends—may mistakenly regard the therapist even more highly for his socializing. That "he's a regular guy" is fine—but not what qualifies the therapist to add to his patient list.

Yet the other side of the coin is even stronger: *Almost every patient wants the therapist to be his personal friend.* "Even among those of us who know that social relationships don't make for good therapeutic relationships, the pressures are tremendous to give in," another shrink explains. "Many patients will do virtually anything for a mere momentary personal exchange with the therapist. I have personally known of a case where the patient invested in a three-thousand-dollar telescope to be able to see when the analyst was leaving his apartment and hopefully bump into him on the street by 'chance.'"

The reason for such behavior is plain: The patient is so completely vulnerable to the therapist. This is the one person, even more than the patient's mate, who knows his fantasies, weaknesses, and deep dark secrets. Always in the back of the patient's mind, therefore, is the question,

"What does he think of me? Does he like me?" And in back of *that* is the wish not only to be liked and appreciated in spite of one's problems, but to be the "favorite patient," to be, in fact, good enough to rate as an equal to the therapist socially.

But filling up one's time and elevating oneself socially are only the outer edge of the abuses of psychotherapy on the part of the patient. There are many wrong reasons to go into therapy. Actually, most people go into most important relationships for the wrong reasons. Those who form relationships for pretty much the right reasons probably don't need therapists. Of course, the therapist theoretically has the unique potential of straightening out a patient who comes to him for the wrong reasons. A woman who appears in a therapist's office because she wants support for something that is patently counterproductive, for example, *may* wind up seeing that she is there for precisely the wrong reason and stays for precisely the right reason.

But not very often.

If you are in psychotherapy or contemplating it, the most important hour, or hours, you can spend will be devoted to knowing exactly *why* you want to go to a therapist.

Chances are you will discover that a therapist is *not* the person you most want to see.

18
Does Hardly Anyone Need Therapy?

Maybe the best case against professional therapy is that comparatively few need it at all.

To the person plagued with problems who just read those words—or who is sympathetic to the masses of human beings with real psychological suffering—the idea may seem cruel and unthinking. But what if it is our unthinking acceptance of therapy that has cruelly exacerbated our suffering? What if we've been brainwashed to buy the idea behind psychoanalysts and psychologists and encounter groups just as we've been sold twenty-four-hour deodorants and feminine "protection" sprays?

One of the happiest, most "adjusted" persons I have ever known is a leading commercial artist who catches rattlesnakes in his spare time. Happily married to a successful fine artist, with four fine sons and a beautiful house of redwood and glass within a small forest, he has always kept himself in excellent physical condition and looks fifteen years younger than he is. Having known him since 1956 without ever once thinking that he didn't smell good, I was more than surprised one day, when the subject of deodorant came up, to hear him remark, "I've never used it." A very inner-directed person, he believed that hardly anyone needed deodorant and that the more you used it, the more you would need it.

What makes us buy commercial deodorant is pretty much what makes us buy commercial therapy. We're too other-people-directed, our most prevalent and painful neurosis being the fear of what *they* will think of us. Even if we smell ok, it *isn't* ok.

But maybe we *do* smell all right. Maybe we seldom if ever need *deodorant.* Maybe it's almost always . . . in our minds.

My grandfather often told the story of the mother who brought to him a young boy who was convinced that a bean had lodged in his rectum. "It's on his mind every waking minute," the mother said hysterically. "You have to do something. I've taken him to see half a dozen psychiatrists!"

My grandfather whispered to his receptionist: "Go to the grocery store on the corner and buy me some beans." After she returned, "Poppa" ushered the boy into his private office, asked him what the problem was, and nodded agreeably when the boy told him. Poppa then, palming a bean, asked the boy to drop his pants, whereupon he examined him and, eureka, produced the bean!

"There it is," Poppa said, "But I'll tell you what we're going to do. We're going to put the bean in this jar" and my grandfather took a sterile jar from his table, dropped the bean in and then turned the lid until it was tight, "so you won't have any more trouble."

The boy was ecstatic. He rushed out into the waiting room to show his mother. My grandfather was behind him, winking at her wisely. She called a week later to say that her son had completely returned to normal. Safely atop his dresser was the jar with the bean inside.

Yes, we all have problems. People have always had problems. Yet people haven't always had professional therapy. Our problems are thousands and thousands of years old, yet therapy is in its infancy. Can anyone honestly say that the world is *less* troubled now than before there were psychoanalysts, psychologists, and encounter groups?

Quite obviously, the opposite is true. We have more problems now than ever before.

Is it because our modern age is so much more difficult in which to live? Even if this *were* true, the very qualities that are characteristic of the twentieth century—a frightening overcomplexity and a threatening inner dependency—are characteristic of therapy. And maybe the best answers are simple ones.

An article entitled "Do You Feel Depressed? You're

Probably Right," in the *Chicago Tribune* of February 15, 1981, gives scientific proof for Thoreau's wise observation that what we think about ourselves truly determines what we feel about others, about life, and our fate. The article cites a study by Lauren B. Alloy, psychologist at Northwestern University, who in conjunction with University of Wisconsin assistant professor Lyn Y. Abramson, decided to test the almost universally accepted idea that if we are depressed, it's because we have the wrong values or a depressed view of life. The implication of such a view, of course, is that therapy can change what we feel and therefore make us less depressed. But what Alloy and Abramson found was that depressed persons may suffer more because they have a rational view of life: "They give themselves credit for both good and bad events." On the other hand, "Nondepressed people may see themselves in a positive light," which may actually be a *real* distortion. But that distortion, though it may not significantly change the actual events in the life of a nondepressed person as compared to a depressed one, makes the one person *less* depressed.

The article notes that other studies have come up with similar results.

Still other studies suggest that, except for almost pathological-like depression that renders an individual nonfunctional, people don't want to change their outlook. They may say they do. The individual who mainly sees the hole in the doughnut will claim he'd like to be a more positive thinker, while the more Pollyannaish person will often want "to try and be realistic." Yet how many people have you known whose basic outlook on life truly changed from childhood? And part of it is that *they don't want to change.* We will generally choose as mates, best friends, or partners people who give us the "other side" so that we can "have" the opposite in a sense without *being* it. Arlo Guthrie, the brilliant and contemplative troubadour and composer (whose performing partner often is the ever-ebullient Pete Seeger), had an insightful line about this in his fine film, *Alice's Restaurant.* It occurs in the subtle but climactic confrontation between Arlo and Alice's husband, Ray, who always wants to be on a "high." He and Alice had been having trouble, so he has a gigantic wedding recelebration, inviting all the younger people with whom he surrounds himself. The party slows a little, though, and Ray begins talking of filling a giant balloon house with helium which they'll all float to the sky and live in. Before leaving, Arlo quietly but profoundly tells him that people don't want to be happy *all* the time.

Even if they wanted to, they can't be. Therapy can help us improve the quality of life, but it cannot change our own basic qualities as individuals. Paul Simon's moving song about a beaten but unbowed boxer superpercep-tively tells us that "after changes we are more or less the same." Yet our longtime Judeo-Christian ethic, combined with a frighteningly complex, pressurized society (which, through mere overpopulation alone, may drive even the

sanest of us mad in the twenty-first century), and cat-
alyzed by our addiction to doctors have made it almost
incumbent upon everyone "to try and change." People
do change: They become more, or less, of what they are
and what they could be. We have free will, but, as Freud
told every future therapist, the decisions we make as
adults are in a sense minor ones. They are all based on
decisions we made unconsciously at what may seem
frighteningly early in life.

Actually, when one stops to think about it, it isn't so
frightening that we made many of those decisions at four
or six or ten. Children, unless emotionally battered from
the outside, usually have much more self-esteem, purity,
and sense of life than adults.

In fact, possibly the most meaningful way to sum up the
simplicity and beauty of children is this: Before a dic-
tatorial or disappointing world shackles or cripples most
of them, they expect the world to be what *they* would
like.

*It is only later that they think of changing to accommo-
date the world.*

19
And Even if You Need Therapy, Do You Want it?

I met a man six years ago who was what might be called an obsessive horseplayer. Because of a pastime we had in common, we'd bump into each other and talk for several minutes every few months about the horses. He was not a gambler per se, he was only interested in horse racing. He loved it.

And he went for it, winning great sums of money, losing great sums of money, going to the track every chance he could, knowing the full range of ecstasy and despair. Even in his worst moments, though, there was always the excitement of tomorrow. He was almost a proselytizer for playing the horses.

His marriage began to suffer as a result. He had sent, or was sending, every one of his children through college, had a nice house and a nice car, and lived in a nice suburb.

When he won, he spent the money, and when he lost, he was under pressure to produce more in his business to take back to the track. A few years ago he began talking about giving it up because his wife was threatening to leave him. I didn't see him until almost two years after that. He greeted me proudly announcing that he hadn't been to the track in almost a year. "And you know what?" he added. "It's amazing how much money I find in my pockets and how many suits of clothes I have in the closet."

"And you have more self-respect, too," I said.

He nodded. "And I have my wife."

It's an exception for me to talk to people at random, even for a few minutes. But this fellow had always been fascinating. Now, I found myself no longer interested in hearing what he had to say. I didn't have an aversion to him; I simply found him boring. *Boring.* He *was* a "better man" for what he'd done. I'm sure he did have more suits in his closet, money in his pocket, and a wife he needed at home. Her dictum and possibly the pressure had done for him what a therapist *might* have been able to accomplish. He felt better about himself in an important way.

And one would think that this would make him happier.

But he seemed distinctly *less* happy. He was more content, more at peace. But he *wasn't* as *happy*.

Because he had lost his one great passion.

This man is not an Edison who has suddenly lost his interest in the electric light, or a Tchaikowsky not even interested in composing the *Pathétique* as his elegy. Yet because he was neither an Edison nor a Tchaikowsky didn't mean he couldn't have one great love, one great passion.

We all do. As with Alan Strang, who was "cured" of his by a compromising therapist in *Equus;* most of us have it parented or cultured or analyzed out of us by the time we are adults. For some who seem blessed,the passion, diffuse though strong at the beginning, survives and takes a tangible form at some later point in our lives.

A famous psychologist once told of a butcher who endured incalculable abuse from his wife over the course of a long marriage. She could say virtually anything, it seemed, and he would take it, night after night, year after year. One evening, they had another couple over for dinner. As he was carving the roast beef, the butcher's wife began abusing him verbally. She said things so cutting that the other man and woman were speechless. Her husband again didn't bat an eyelash. But then she climaxed a particularly abusive string of invectives with, "You can't even carve a roast beef after twenty years as a butcher."

She had never said *that* to him before. He dropped the carving knife and the fork, went into the basement and got his suitcase, packed and left the house without a word, never to return.

I love that butcher.

Neurosis, of course, need not be one great passion or pride in something. Neurosis may take itself out in a thousand forms. *Genuinely* crazy people are pretty boring and fall into markedly similar groups; they may make the headlines by killing someone or standing naked at the top of a building and threatening to jump, but it is only because these actions are so antisocial, not because of their uniqueness, that they make headlines. A couple of years ago I was offered the chance to do a book on John Wayne Gacy, the part-time clown who murdered dozens of children. I would have access to unpublished information on the case and to *him* in his cell. I turned it down without a second thought. Above and beyond the fact that I wouldn't want to spend my time writing about such a subhuman, I knew he wouldn't have interested me nearly as much as the butcher who had the discipline and the value system to take virtually any kind of abuse for twenty years, but wouldn't take a crucial kind for twenty seconds. For whatever form neurosis takes, it is distinctly *human.* And in the end it always orbits around some price we personally pay, in the widest sense some pain we suffer, to gain something of value to us. There is no such thing as a free lunch. The John Gacys cannot carve a roast beef skillfully; they can only stick knives in people's backs. It takes no discipline or humanity for them to live with what they do, and, if they are made to pay the proper price by society, it is the one price above all a neurotic wants to avoid paying.

Neurotics—human beings—see therapists either because they would like their suffering diminished or because they want to free themselves to carve their particular roast beef better. If the therapist can help them to see their situation and themselves more clearly, they may suffer more productively, but there will still be suffering in life—in a life worth living. The price of something worthwhile is always how much it takes to acquire and keep it. If, on the other hand, their therapy results in their *caring less* about what really matters to them, they become to a degree like the other side of Gacy coin—less caring "pods." The motion picture *Invasion Of The Body Snatchers* so acutely delineated this, and Ira Levin carried it to its logical extension in *The Stepford Wives.*

When therapy can treat you so that you can live better with your neuroses, fine. But don't treat your neuroses lightly. Actually, what therapy can best do is to make you *value them.* They may be what is most worthwhile about you; they are inextricably bound to all human achievement and love, as well as what makes you most interesting and unique as a human being.

And because they are distinctly human—dogs and other pets can become neurotic to a degree, because they live with people—neuroses are inherently dignifying. And inevitable. I have met only a handful of individuals in my life who, without therapy, were without any significant neurosis. I admit to not knowing them very well. What's to know?

Most of us, however, because we have a deep need for acceptance at almost any price, are often unlike the heroine of *The Fantasticks,* who prayed to God not to let her be normal because she wanted "much more." We curb our aspirations and tranquilize our passions, bury our fears and cremate our ecstasies.

There is the story of a man who goes to a therapist three times a week for almost five years. In that time he reveals a huge amount about himself, to which the psychiatrist answers with questions such as, "Why do you feel that?" or "What do you feel when you say that?" or simply nods or stares.

Finally, the patient becomes fed up. "I've been paying you $35 a session three times a week for almost five years," he shouts angrily. "And you haven't once given even the slightest hint as to what my problem might be!"

"Oh, I know what your problem is," the therapist answers.

"Then why didn't you say anything all this time?" the man bellows.

"You didn't ask me," the therapist replies.

"Well what *is* my problem?"

"You're in love with your raincoat," the therapist answers coolly.

The patient explodes. "In love with my *raincoat.* In love with my *raincoat!* How can you *say* such a *stupid* thing? For five years I've been coming here three times a week, revealing all my emotional complexities, and now all you can tell me is that I'm in love with my raincoat? I'm going to *sue* you! I'm going to have you disbarred! I'm—"

The therapist holds up his hand. "Now hold on a minute," he says. "If I ask you one question, do you promise to give me an honest answer? Because this one question can solve everything."

"Sure, I'll answer honestly. But it won't change how angry I am at that ridiculous thing you said."

"OK," the therapist says quietly. "Now answer honestly: Do you or do you not love your raincoat?"

The patient wrinkles his brow and wrings his hands in disgust. "No," he says emphatically, "I do not love my raincoat." Then, "Friends? Yes. But love? Never."

The story is apocryphal, but the point is not. The point is: Talking to your raincoat is obviously a delusional sign of psychosis. We can afford to joke about it only because the joke isn't personally hurtful to the psychotic; he's laughing at you because he thinks *you're* crazy for *not* having a relationship with *your* raincoat.

And seldom can a therapist substantively change that.

Ayn Rand had a beautiful passage in *The Fountainhead* about how people compromise and change and call it growth. The hero of that novel never changes, nor should he.

Nor, in the deepest sense, should we.

There is an absolute distinction, and one that has been lost among most of us lately, between using our enormous free will to change our lives and *changing*. Even the briefest look at history shows that those whose goal it was to change the world or its people have made most of the trouble for the rest of us. Many people did change the world and made life better for us, however, by *doing*, unchangingly, what they had always done best. Edison wasn't trying to change the world, only sit in his laboratory and create light. Because of him we don't live in darkness.

Apply it to yourself, Look back over your life, with a hard honesty, and see if it isn't the accommodations you made that brought you trouble. Throw off for a golden moment the unquestioned, suffocating, and cynical demand that we change to accommodate others, the world, or somebody's idea of what is best.

That idea is usually the *only* one worth changing.

20
Why Therapy Can Kill Creativity

In July 1980 Walter Cronkite presented a report on an "enchanted" youngster named Nadia, who, at six, began producing drawings so boggling in their beauty and technique that art teachers and museum directors judged them "genius." But because of her autism—which Cronkite wisely described as behavior that psychiatrists don't know how to explain—therapists tried to "help" the child. By *their* standards, they did. Yet as her behavior became more and more like that of the rest of us, her drawings became more and more like those the rest of us would produce. By the time she was twelve, this enchanted girl with genius was well on her way toward being just about the same as everyone else, her drawings worthy more of her family's kitchen wall.

This is a familiar unfamiliar story. Unfamiliar, because

few of us are born with such talent. Familiar, because therapy is inherently at odds with creative genius. Therapists, on the whole, "treat" the aberrant behavior of the artist as if it were neurotic or counterproductive. Since the quality of art is always arguable, one can measure therapy's success or failure only by how productive the artist is after therapy.

Though there are notable examples of writers, painters, composers producing more after seeing a shrink, most often the creative person becomes *less* creative after seeing a psychiatrist. The equation is a simple one: The artist suffers; he bears that suffering, even makes it into ecstasy, by subliminating it into art; remove much of the suffering and you remove the need to subliminate it.

There were great artists for thousands of years before there were therapists. It is questionable how many great artists, if any, we have had in the several decades since formal therapy has become established. What is the therapist's answer to this? Usually, the therapist answers that the artist of today who so frequently goes into therapy suffers less, and is better adjusted as a result.

Many "creative" patients of therapists agree. It has frequently been observed that possibly the greatest curse is to possess something of the aspiration or the vision while possessing only *something* of the talent to back it up. For such a writer or artist or composer therapy *can* be a temporary way out of a dilemma. What marks the artist as different from the rest of us is his talent to feel more intensely about things, and in this intensity see a larger picture or details of the picture with a perception the rest of us lack. He expresses what he sees not primarily in relationships with other human beings but in his relationship with the reality he perceives.

If a true artist can accomplish this, an unsurpassed ecstasy is the reward. Even so, particularly as mortality increasingly stares him in the face, he may increasingly opt to taste and feel the reality around him that binds him to others rather than the reality within his mind. Woody Allen once said incisively that he didn't want immortality in his work, he wanted it in his life. It takes grit, as well as genius, to remain an artist until the end. But if you are *not*, if year after year passes without a significant sign that your work will achieve any immortality, you begin desperately to need what is available to you as a mortal man. The life scenarios of the greatest artists are frequently punctuated by escapes into alcoholism, drugs, breakdowns, chaotic love affairs, suicidal attempts. To the would-be-but-not-truly-creative individual such escape is optional. The tunnel vision of the creative genius is tunneled into *his* vision. The would-be can return to the world, and probably should. For him therapy *is* an opiate. He can go into intensive analysis for a few years or merely visit a psychologist for a few months and come out saying what one *fairly* successful writer confided to me (almost a paraphrase of what hundreds of other moderately accomplished people in the arts have told me): "I struggled for years—for what? My therapist showed me an alternative. I can write now without approaching writing as if it were my whole life. I've learned to do and enjoy so many things I never did before. You ought to go see him." Sooner or later, however, in almost every case, the creative output of such patients drops. They spend more time relating to others, make some major move—a new job, a new house—that further assimilates them into the world from which they once existed essentially apart. Within a few years they only dabble at what once was the purpose of their lives, saying they are more content this way, or are laying the groundwork to going back into creative endeavors full time. That day rarely comes. Instead they tend increasingly to show their friends what they *have* done or talk to them about it rather than *doing* it. The would-be artist is now a "might-have-been." Or is it a "should-be" that never was?

But not when it is based on a lie. Better if they faced themselves squarely and said, "I don't have the talent or the dedication, I'm going to do something else"—or even, "I'm just not extreme enough to be a real artist. I want to enjoy what other people enjoy without all that struggle." Yet the therapist seldom confronts them with whether they have what it takes or whether they want it badly enough. Instead, he tends to provide a sounding board for the half-truths they have been uttering to themselves: "Real quality can't make it in this world" — "I owe it to my family" — "I can't create with these pressures hanging over me" — "I'll get back to it when the time is right" — "My hemorrhoids are bothering me."

The shrink has a vested interest in seeing these people changed. They aren't going to make it. They are suffering for nothing. Better that they should lose the suffering and gain some enjoyment—and sing the shrink's praises. *He* wants success, too.

But the vested interest of the therapist in the would-be artist's becoming a "full person" is nothing compared with his interest in the genuine artist. Here the therapist is more than a sounding board; he would become the board of directors. Or a *partner* . . . in art . . . as if there could ever be such a thing. Down deep, he wants the artist to stay in therapy at almost any cost. Why?

First, because the true artist is interesting. By definition, such a patient is unique, far more entertaining, indeed, than the ordinary neurotics the therapist must confront hour after hour, day in and day out. The artist may have the same basic problems as any other patient, but through what he is they metamorphose into something infinitely more engaging. Did he have a domineering, guilt-giving mother? If so, maybe he is thinking of sleeping with her. Or killing her. Or . . . writing a book about sleeping with her or killing her. His neuroses are *transformed,* because they are *part* of his *art.* As one of the two best editors with whom I ever worked told me when I began my first novel: "You're risking your life. If you don't do it, or if it's no good, you won't be able to say,

'I had a difficult childhood, my wife and I weren't getting along, my ulcer put me in the hospital.' Because all of that has to go into your novel."

Thus, a second reason shrinks are drawn to artists is that the *artist* is actually a *model* for *the therapist*. The artist has problems, the artist suffers, the artist may go to the shrink because of it. But precisely because everything in the artist's life is subsumed into his art, he has it all "together." He may even write a play about the therapist. And the therapist wouldn't mind that at all.

Yet, for the psychotherapist, the most compelling pull to the artist (and generally to *any* celebrity or individual or sizable dedication and accomplishment) is that many a therapist is himself a would-have-been artist. Do you really believe that the tweedy, rational fellow sitting across from you doesn't have fantasies? Wouldn't like to be a star? Doesn't want to produce something more lasting than an adjusted accountant?

Thus, the therapist is generally involved—*too* involved, because *any* personal involvement is too much—with the creative achiever. Not only may the therapist glory vicariously in his identification with the patient's creative efforts, but there is potential reflected glory for him should those efforts "succeed." The actress or the writer who is temporarily "helped" by a therapist will probably either talk about it publicly or express it in his work. A notable example of someone who has sung the praises of his therapy is film-maker Woody Allen, who has said publicly that therapy helped him enormously. And therapy *does* help a small number of artists enormously, at least in the short run. Yet these questions must be asked before the final verdict is in.

First: How can an artist be sure that he would not have been equally as productive and brilliant if he had not gone into therapy, if he had sought out some other catalyst for whatever he felt was stopping him from doing the most he could? Second, while one cannot argue with results, a key question is *what the long-range results of therapy* will be. Whether or not one thinks Woody Allen is funny or incisive, whether or not one likes his films, is subjective. Whatever they are, let us see how strongly they continue to flow from him. It *could* be, of course, that Allen has one of those rare therapists who is himself an artist. It *could* be that Allen is one of those rare people who can take what he needs from therapy and cast aside all that is unnecessary or dangerous.

But most true artists, like most people, cannot do so. If the artist mistakenly goes to the therapist for artistic problems—say, he is temporarily blocked or continuously pays some heavy price for his creative production—how in the world is a therapist qualified to help? Every artist is "blocked" during some period of his life. Katherine Anne Porter took well over a decade to write *Ship of Fools.* Would it have been a better book—would it ever have been a book—if she had seen a therapist after six arduous years? Thank goodness there was no formal field of psychiatry during Thoreau's time! I can just see a shrink saying to him, "Don't you think going off to Walden Pond is a regression?" Of all the human achievements, with the possible exception of the true love relationship, nothing is more evanescent, more subjectively complex, than giving birth to an enduring work of art. No scientific discipline can capture it.

And what if the artist sees a therapist for personal, human problems that plague him, even though he is, all in all, producing his best creatively? If the therapist is not able to help him, the therapy has failed. If the therapist is able to help him, the therapy may succeed, but the artist fail. Yes, the artist may find more pleasure and contentment in life through better relationships, more creature comforts, less self-destructive impulses, or whatever the therapist is able to give him as a human being. But in the majority of cases this pulls the artist further away from his center. Contentment, yes. Pleasure, yes, Adjustment, yes. Comfort, yes. But happiness? How can the true artist be happier when part of his purpose is committed to his "ordinary" self? Frequently, Tchaikovsky, a homosexual, vowed an attempt to be "normal." During each such episode he produced less. And, though formal therapy is relatively recent, there has always been *therapy*. Van Gogh desperately opted for it when he went to live with Gauguin, and that episode may well have marked Vincent's downward turning point.

Professional therapy has marked the downward turning point for a number of twentieth-century artists. For psychotherapy can be a more potent "remedy" than cocaine and alcohol together. The artist will at least pass out when he has drunk too much, ruin his nostrils after snorting too much cocaine. Too much therapy seldom gives us any physical warnings.

During the few months that I saw a therapist a few years ago, because I wanted to learn firsthand what my wife had considered such a vital experience for her, there was one revealing discussion. It was virtually the only revealing discussion I had with him. It revealed something about him, not about me. I had begun to feel there was nothing important for me to find with a psychotherapist, and the session came to the point where we actually began arguing about whether or not this was true. Naturally, the therapist's pat answer is usually that you get out of something what you put into it and that the patient isn't trying hard enough or his motives aren't genuine enough if therapy doesn't help him. But I refused to have the ball always thrown back to me, and told this dear analytic Brutus that the fault might not lie in his patients but in himself—or, most of all, in the inherent nature of psychotherapy being a creative personality's antipode. And that, in fact, "adjustment" was anathema to creativity.

"Nonsense," he replied smoothly. "Many great artists have been very well adjusted."

"Name one," I said.

"Rubens."

After a week of thinking about his answer, and of looking into biographical data on Rubens, I realized I had been bluffed in a game of psychiatric poker by a jack when I had a king showing and held all the aces. I began the next session, then, by asking to see the analyst's hole card—or *any* other card: "Can you name another besides Rubens?"

He didn't.

There are no doubt well-adjusted artists and writers and composers of note.

But not many.

Even if you count Rubens.

There was a time when I could not understand the absolute truth and wisdom of the story—and I have read much the same story a hundred times over—of the older critic at a party who spots a young novelist whose brilliant first work she has recently read. The critic immediately goes over to the writer, thinking of the best way to express what she feels for the artist's work. "You don't know what you've done," she says simply.

The artist does not know how he produces his most original work. It's like falling in love. I have personally experienced this with the one novel among my forty-five books. I tried every way I knew how to write it, and couldn't. Because I didn't know how. Then, when I was thirty-seven, I stopped trying to learn how, and it wrote itself for me.

We are surrounded by a world so dehumanized that even the word *dehumanized* is plastic.

Possibly its sickest symptom is that the computer and those measurers who run it are everywhere, like the Lilliputians tying down Gulliver, telling us that if we will only answer these fifty-seven questions, we will find out what Heinz variety of talent we have. Sad. To have to take a test to find out what your gifts are!

Capabilities scream to be used, from early childhood onward. The ultra-plastic presumption that we need to take tests to find out what we would love to do is father to the stillborn notion that we need treatment to use our gifts properly. It is like a sex manual for the soul.

And the contradiction between creativity and psychotherapy holds meaning for all of us. Because there is an artist within all of us, though we may not all be artists or pursue any form of creativity as our profession.

The meaning is this: If you are fortunate enough and gritty enough to survive as an adult having something that you *absolutely love to do* . . . do it.

Don't analyze it.

21
When Therapy Works –
The Patient as Therapist

All of this is not to say that therapy always fails. Even when the therapist is not a skilled artist at his craft, therapy sometimes works and helps the patient more than it hurts. Especially when therapy is short term, it frequently does less harm than good for any number of reasons, such as the fact that even with a poor therapist, now and then the chemistry is right between him and certain patients. Or, in crisis therapy, *anyone* who listens, and seems to be calm and empathic, will probably help.

Yet both of these situations underscore that the *patient sometimes becomes the therapist.*

The TV show "Maude" had an episode illustrating this point. The overbearing, strident, very verbal Maude had enough of a problem to make her seek out a therapist for a single session. The therapist is never seen by the viewer, and never heard. Because Maude walks in, begins talking about the problem, voices the alternatives herself, expresses her feelings, and works the whole thing out by the end of the session. Yet maybe the most profound line is when she rises to leave, gratefully thanking the therapist for giving her the solution to the problem!

Talking out loud to oneself has been ridiculed and stigmatized by society, but it is usually nothing more, or nothing less, than thinking out loud. So few of us ever acquire the habit of sitting down and thinking out our problems at all that to think out loud seems laughable or schizophrenic. Nothing could be further from the truth. This is why we have long had the apocryphal story of the philosopher who, when questioned by a skeptical bystander about why he talked to himself so much, answered: "Because I want an intelligent conversation."

Try it sometime. You will not only have an intelligent conversation, but one with the person most interested in you and, increasingly, who knows you best. You will find that, without a therapist, you are usually able to do what Maude did, which was the whole point of what Maude did. And you will save yourself the economic burden, rigidity of schedule, time, and everything else that is required in therapy.

It is not only a matter of the psychotherapeutic process being crucially dependent upon the patient. It is again what Thoreau said at the outset of *Walden*—that he would be writing in the first person and talking about his own experiences because he was more interested in and knew more about them than anything else.

If we stop ... and think ... most of us would be surprised at how much we indeed do know about ourselves.

22
The Best Defense is a Good Defense

In 1971 I wrote my first novel, *She Lives!* It was the story of two teen-agers madly in love. Shortly after they began living together, they discover that the girl has an incurable cancer. Instead of accepting that the cancer is incurable and taking Pam for treatment, Andy devotes every hour to finding a *cure.* At the eleventh hour he discovers a brilliant researcher in another part of the country who has had experimental success with what was then a radical form of treatment: autoimmunology. Andy and Pam travel to the doctor's clinic and, against all odds, convince him to experiment with her. Within a short time the cancer is gone for good.

Autoimmunology, the science of supporting and stimulating the body's natural defenses, *our immune system* that kills off attackers from cancer to the common cold, may be the key to psychological and physiological health.

Medical science in the past decade has come to realize and demonstrate convincingly that, through the body's natural defenses, we are killing off cancer cells virtually all the time. It is only when our defenses are dangerously weakened or crippled by consistent abuse, such as the smoking of cigarettes, by traumatic abuse, as with an overwhelming overdose of radiation, or by the abuse of time itself that a cancer can take hold. Otherwise, to the fully healthy *inner* body an assault by cancer cells may be merely sport for an immunological system, and often strengthen that system because it can use the exercise. This is why the bodies of prisoners who volunteer to be implanted with cancer reject malignant cells. On the other hand, if you inject cancer cells into someone who has had cancer, even if that cancer is seemingly arrested or eradicated by some such external weapon as surgery, chemicals, or whatever, the malignant tumor will usually "take." This may also explain why so many patients with a seemingly controlled or eradicated cancer develop a new malignancy in some seemingly unrelated site.

This applies equally to any illness. At the other end of the continuum from cancer, for example, is the common cold. We may well discover some day that the same virus that often produces sniffles can, in a person with far less immunological defense, produce a cancer. But where our body will call out all the troops when confronted by cancer cells, it rightly does not react the same to the common cold. We will kill off the cold, which is why no one has a cold forever, but only by employing relatively few physiological infantrymen rather than our nuclear capabilities. And because our autoimmune system is not truly threatened by a cold, nearly everyone gets colds. Integral to the automatic "wisdom" of our natural ammunition system is that it will not waste itself on clay pigeons.

But what if a cold consistently turns into pneumonia? Sometimes, it *may,* if our immunological system has been weakened to *that* level. And what if the pneumonia were to kill us if not treated by antibiotics and the like? Then that is because our immunological system is at a *crucially* low level. Sure, we should take the antibiotic and save our lives. But we should know that *as long as our immunological system is at a level where it would permit our death from some outside invader, we are prey to all kinds of other diseases, because our health is in a state of Russian roulette.* Yes, we may be saved again and again by outside intervention, but it is a perilous and certainly not a healthfully autonomous existence—and inevitably it is not as long an existence.

Because the brain, in its capacity *not* to act automatically, differs radically from the rest of the body, we overlook the even more important similarity between brain and body: Both are made up of cells and fundamentally subject to the same physiological principles. Possibly the most important of those principles is the *defense mechanism.*

Whatever ways in which the many forms of therapy differ, *all have in common the necessity to break down some defenses of the patient.*

On the face of it, it would seem, then, that therapy is absurd and destructive. Therapists tell us that the goal is to knock down the defenses that aren't productive and keep intact as much as possible those that are. They tell us that a defense that is less than ideal can be destroyed and built anew more rationally. They may even say, as electroshock therapists who erased part of our memories said a generation ago, that intense or prolonged types of therapy indeed do act as chemotherapy does on cancer (though hopefully "only" no more drastically than an antibiotic).

But logic says otherwise, as does patient after patient I have personally seen. After therapy, though knowing more in certain ways about themselves and adjusting better to others, they are less happy and less truly secure, and have marked changes in their lives or in their personalities *not* for the better.

That we have become willing to allow therapy, both in practice and in its wider influence, to batter down our psychological immune system, is nowhere plainer than in our current cultural catchwords: "Don't be defensive!" *Vulnerability,* a term derived from unprotectedness and weakness in battle (and, by implication, the battle of life) now has a positive connotation in the psychological sense that contradicts the physiologically negative connotation.

We have our defenses for a reason. Unless we are suffering such severe anguish that we must have our defenses broken down in order to extricate the pain, the weight of logic and the bulk of evidence strongly suggest that destroying defenses is more harmful than getting to the problems in back of them. The epigraph of Robert Ruark's insightful novel, *Something Of Value,* warns that if we would break down someone's traditions, customs, and daily pleasures, we had better replace them with something of value. Therapy, even not-so-good therapy, does give us something—a different way of looking at things, self-knowledge, someone who will listen when we talk. But are those things of enough value when weighed against the destruction of our defenses?

Therapy by nature carries a big stick. How often can it truly speak softly?

As a matter of fact, our physiological immunity indeed seems startlingly dependent upon the extent of our psychological invulnerability. In *She Lives!* the onset of Pam's cancer occurs shortly after she undergoes a trauma with which she cannot cope: the accidental death of her brother and parents. Studies in a leading New York research hospital, among others, reveal that an overwhelming majority of first-time cancer patients report an "irreplaceable loss" in their lives within eighteen months preceding the diagnosis of the tumor. One man's irreplaceable loss, of course, is merely another man's difficult situation. I have known men who hated their work and looked forward to retirement, and who prospered because the hobbies they pursued in their retirement were the work they should have been doing. More often, I have seen vigorous men whose careers were suddenly taken away by forced retirement (or by their own mistaken idea that they should retire and "take it easy") immediately fall prey to strokes, accidents, heart attacks, or, within a year or so, cancer. I have watched young athletes who took bone-breaking punishment without so much as complaining. Yet, when cut from the team, slip on the sidewalk and fracture their legs. In fact, never have I seen a person lose someone on something about which he cared deeply without his health soon suffering in some severe, though hopefully temporary, way. When the someone or something of value that is lost is the most important thing in life and cannot be replaced, I have seldom seen survivors.

The classic psychological example of a person with virtually no defenses, is the schizophrenic. In *The Denial of Death*, Ernest Becker says: "The schizophrenic feels these [dreads of death and of the overwhelmingness of life] more than anyone else because he hasn't been able to build the confident defenses that a person normally uses to deny them."

Vulnerable is . . . *vulnerable.*

23
You Cannot Treat the Untreatable

Once again, despite therapy's inherent deficiencies and injurious assumptions, a number of therapists—and their patients—overcome. But just as there are "problems" for which you ought not go to a therapist, there are "problems" for which you *cannot* go to a therapist.

In the months before Dr. Gelperin had his heart attack he and Anne talked about sometime talking about her absolute fear of death. Like Anne, Gelperin said he hated death, though had none of the overwhelming fear of it that Anne and I harbor.

A surpassingly down-to-earth man, he would have been attempting the impossible to free Anne of her fear. It is grimly revealing that he did not live long enough to try and "help" her deal with this "problem." Had he lived to be ninety, however, nothing he could have said would have allayed her fear one iota.

Anne and I are absolutely afraid of death because it is *the* absolute that inextricably stands against life. No matter what pain and problems we have had, we cannot for an instant, with the least amount of equanimity, imagine that some day we wouldn't *be* here, wouldn't *know*, wouldn't be *aware*, wouldn't have a *tomorrow*. We have felt this from our very early childhood when it first dawned on us that there is such a thing as death. It was the most significant trauma in both our lives. When we later examined our fear, it seemed not only supra rational, but the basis for all rationality. The more one wants or treasures the joy of life, the more one would fear and hate no life.

Otto Rank said that to confront full-on the time limit of life *without* extreme anxiety is impossible. In any event, we are all, at best, individuals and have individual ways of dealing with death and with the dark side of life. Despite the price paid by Anne and myself because of our inability and unwillingness to accept the fact that we will die, our hate and fear of death is necessary to the core of our lives.

We are untreatable.

Because death is untreatable. And for every person there are sacred and profane untreatables. Alfred Adler advised "[any therapist] who has acquired this much insight will refrain from undertaking . . . tedious excursions into mysterious regions of the psyche." This is not to affirm Kierkegaard's belief that the opiate to confronting death fully is a tranquilizing with the trivial. No lesson has come boomeranging back on us more dramatically in this final quarter of the twentieth century than that we should not ignorantly attempt to manipulate nature. Nor can we ever learn the truths of nature and of survival for our planet if our unquestioned axiom is to manipulate our own natures?

The most meaning-filled short story I have ever encountered is Nathaniel Hawthorne's "The Birthmark," the tale of a brilliant scientist whose life is incomplete because he does not have the perfect woman to love. Lo and behold, he finds her—perfect in every respect for him, with the single small exception of a tiny birthmark, almost like the tip of a finger lightly touching her cheek. The birthmark begins to obsess him because she is so perfect otherwise, and he turns all his scientific endeavors toward finding some formula that will remove it. Time and again he fails, but ultimately he comes up with something that indeed removes the tiny, light spot! Once it is gone, she dies.

The removing of all our birthmarks is not noble. It is the *easy* way, born of the lack of courage to *recognize* what we are and of the grit to *be* what we are. Turn on the TV, open a newspaper, or simply look around you. Has something gone wrong? The government will make it right. You have a headache? If the pill with three ingredients doesn't do the trick, then try the one with four. Does death deeply disturb you? Your friendly therapist will fix it. It's all in how you look at it.

But it *isn't.* It is, first and foremost, *what* you're looking at.

We have made an unsavory, dangerous mistake in ignorantly wishing that the same medical means that have increased the length of life can also increase its quality. And because we live longer with so little quality to our lives, the torture builds up all the more until it seems intolerable. We have implored our therapists to become witch doctors, and they have willingly put on the paint and done the dance.

24
Therapy is Dangerous to Us All

You don't have to be a patient—or the mate or business partner, parent or child of a patient—to be hurt by psychotherapy. It is more than possible, for example, that a vital factor in John Lennon's death was the insidious influence psychotherapy has had on the strange permissiveness of our society. And for every John Lennon, there are thousands and thousands of anonymous victims, victims not necessarily of murder, but of the quality of their lives.

An Associated Press release in 1981 reads: "A 55-year-old woman, convicted of first degree murder because she did not try to stop her son from killing his wife, has been sentenced to life in prison . . . [Her son] has acknowledged the slaying, but has pleaded innocent by reason of insanity."

This is more than society's verdict. It is psychotherapy's verdict.

Psychotherapy has adversely affected the lives of all of us. If you are a patient, it may help you or, too often, damage you. If you are not in therapy, though you most certainly escape the dangers inherent in personally seeing a shrink, you can at best *only limit* the harmful side effects from the world around you psychotherapy has produced. By far the most harmful, sometimes fatal, side effect of psychotherapy on society is the concept of *legal* insanity.

Think about that term for a moment.

Legally . . . insane.

What does it mean? For one thing, it means that our system of justice, and the moral beliefs that underlie the government, have been radically altered. For the worse.

What does it mean to you and to me?

It means that thousands and thousands of potential violent acts will become actualized because the courts treat (yes, *treat*) the perpetrators as *temporarily* insane. As *temporary* criminals. Often, the worse the crime, the more this new concept applies, and the more lenient the sentence.

It means that a new generation of Americans has been raised in an atmosphere where insanity resulting in antisocial acts is condoned, or at least dealt with as a psychological aberration instead of a crime.

It means that, for any of us who give any credence to the precept of temporary insanity, our *own* ability to stay sane in times of stress is eroded.

It means much more. One blatant example is overflowing mental institutions that allow the truly destructive personality who should be there for life to walk the streets within months or years, while not spending enough time on those who can hurt only themselves once they are thrown out into society. Those of us who are not in mental institutions are much the worse for this.

First, we are all candiates as victims of brutal, too often lethal, attack by these "alumni" of mental institutions. Second, when we ourselves have emotional problems, we are at the mercy of a view of sanity and morality that is insane and immoral. As Dr. Thomas Szasz said in *Omni* magazine: "The view that the 'mentally ill' person is helplessly in the grip of an 'illness' that 'causes' him to display abnormal behavior is false. Although 'mentally ill' persons may not consciously choose their symptoms, their behavior is, nonetheless, *conduct.*" Szasz quotes G. K. Chesterton's insight that "The last thing that could be said of a lunatic is that his actions are causeless. . . . The madman is not the man who has lost his reason. The madman is the man who has lost everything except his reason." Szasz says that "Such an explanation is too simple and too painful for modern man."

Whether one looks upon insanity as reason devoid of emotion, or emotion devoid of reason, it is insane to look upon insanity as a thing of mood or of the moment. Such a hideous concept robs *sanity* of *everything.*

Sanity, if it has *any* meaning for most of us, is, on the

bottom line, control of our impulses. Not control that stops us from losing our temper and banging our fists on the wall or losing our balance and breaking down in tears. But it does prevent us from hitting a young child instead of a wall, and from descending into a permanent depression instead of a few hours or days of grief or despair. For sanity is not something you move in and out of any more than you move back and forth between life and death. Therapy has fostered such an idea—the monstrous idea of *temporary* insanity.

It is probably the most criminal idea of the twentieth century. An apocryphal story illustrates this.

A reporter was visiting a mental institution for the severely insane to study conditions there. He noticed that one of the patients was following him at a discreet distance. When the reporter was alone, the patient, who appeared in all respects normal enough, approached him.

"I know what you think," the man said. "If I'm in here, I must be crazy. I don't blame you for thinking that. But I heard that you're a reporter, and please, please, hear me out for just half a minute. I promise you it'll be worth your while."

The reporter told the man to go ahead.

"I'm *not* insane," the man began. "I was railroaded in here by my wife and brother. They did it to get control of my fortune. I'm worth several million dollars. I managed to smuggle in papers to prove it—just let me go to my room and bring them to you. *Please.*"

The reporter was beginning to get interested, though still skeptical. "Go ahead," he said. "I'll wait right here."

Within a couple of minutes, the patient returned with an envelope full of letters and legal documents. "Here," he said, handing them to the reporter. "Just take a look."

The reporter looked them over, and was impressed by their evident validity. It did seem that indeed the man had been railroaded into the mental institution so that his wife and brother could get hold of his money.

"Well, was I telling the truth?" the patient asked. "Now do you think I'm crazy or a victim of a terrible injustice?"

"You're definitely not crazy," the reporter answered. "This is one of the worst things I've ever seen. I'm going to write this up for my paper if you let me take these documents back with me."

Tears filled the patient's eyes. "Excuse me . . . For becoming emotional. But you don't know what it's like in here. For six months, it's been living hell. I didn't think I had a chance, then when I heard them talking about you today, I began hoping again. I don't think I could have stood the disappointment if you hadn't listened to me. I'll give you any amount of money you ask for helping me get out of here."

"I don't want any money for it," the reporter said. "It's my job to set wrongs right. I'm going right back to the paper now and write up your story. It should be in Saturday's edition."

"Could I ask you for just one more thing?" the man pleaded.

"Sure, what is it?"

"Now that I know I'll be free soon, I wonder if you'd bring me the paper when it's published. We're not allowed anything like that in here. I only want to see it in print, so that I can know I'll be free for certain soon."

"The Saturday edition comes out at 10:00 A.M.," the reporter said. "I'll be here by noon with it."

The patient grasped the reporter's hand with both of his. "I can't thank you enough. You'll never know—"

"You don't have to thank me," the reporter said, and turned to leave.

Before he'd walked twenty steps, the reporter was struck a hard blow with a brick on the back of the head and fell to his knees. As he tried to rise, he heard the patient saying, "Now don't forget Saturday!"

Why do we laugh? We laugh first, as with almost all effective humor, because we are surprised. And what surprises us in this case is that a seemingly rational person, with whom we identify because he has been unfairly thrust into a totally irrational environment, is suddenly revealed as absolutely, unequivocally nuts. Really crazy. Bonkers. Even with all the trappings of rationality, and an envelope of documents to prove it, the moment he threw that brick we realized he will probably *always* throw that brick and that he likely belongs where he is.

Such insanity seems almost ludicrous to us. And it

159

should seem so. It is something we virtually never run across in our daily lives, something that TV almost never depicts, since it is so far off the beaten human path. On the other hand, when we hear of a Mark David Chapman traveling thousands of miles to gun down John Lennon in front of his New York apartment, John Wayne Gacy shrewdly murdering and burying almost three dozen young boys over a period of years we cannot laugh. We are aghast, so aghast that our common reaction is, "How could they *do* it?"

The question is rhetorical. We *know* how they can do such a thing. Because inside each of us . . . is a murderer. But *we* have not set the murderer free.

Therapy is now setting the murderers free.

25
There is Therapy – and There is Therapy

Two women who have never met before find themselves alone together in the sauna of a health club. They are very different. One is in her forties, fifty pounds overweight, highly intelligent and educated. The other is twenty, not perceptive, and desperately needs to start a dominating conversation. The older woman is a good listener, and the conversation moves from the outside to the inside.

"You see, my father used to hit me. So I got married when I was seventeen to get away from him, but my husband turned out to be the same way. He hit me all the time. I got divorced, and I met Ed. He said he'd never hit me, but I couldn't believe him. It's like every man I'd known had hit me. But it's been a year now, and I know he won't. He's the kind of person who just wouldn't ever hit anyone," the young woman says.

"I was divorced three years ago," the older woman says. "But the stepfather of my children is completely different from my first husband."

"Right. Anyway, we couldn't figure out where to get married. My parents were very religious, and I kind of am too. But he comes from this small town, and we thought a church wedding there would be real decent. I'm taking off four days from work, and we're going to drive there and spend two days and I'll meet everybody he knows."

"Sounds like fun. Coming here is about the only vacation I get these days, with his three kids and my two."

"This'll be my first vacation in a year. We've talked about everything so many times, and I think we're going to get along. He's the kind of person who just would never hit me, you know?"

They talk on. The younger woman keeps coming back to the same thing, the fact that she's sure that the man she's marrying will never be physically violent to her. The older woman talks about a number of things briefly, from her overweight to her new husband's attitude toward the children. After about twenty minutes one of them leaves, pauses at the door to talk for a minute more. They may well bump into each other again, but not necessarily. Still, the encounter has been meaningful, in terms of their daily lives. For they have each given something to one other.

What they have given is . . . therapy.

Any medicine—particularly the potent medicine of psychotherapy's failure—has good side effects as well as bad. The bad may outweigh the good, as with the doctor who advised the patient with a cold to take a warm shower in the middle of winter and then stick his head out the window because, "Sure, you'll have pneumonia now, and that's worse. But we can cure pneumonia—we don't have a cure for the common cold."

The single best side effect of professional therapy's inability to cope is that nonprofessional therapy has burgeoned anew. Throughout virtually every nook and cranny of America there now runs a continuum of "therapy" ranging from the most highly structured groups to the most informal, accidental, one-on-one encounters. Look around and in one direction you will see a plethora of community therapy groups, for example, which have never been there before. Look in the other direction any you will see ordinary people in ordinary life situations putting lay therapeutic techniques that they have learned to use.

Within the next generation, in fact, we may see a revolution in therapy—where those who care for you, *care* for you, where therapy is most often given by those who are not professional therapists, and who identify much more closely with the patient than a therapist. As Dr. Leonard Borman, of Northwestern University's Center for Urban Affairs and director of the Center's Self-Help Institute, says: "The swift growth of the self-help movement is the second Copernican revolution. It shatters the myth of the professional as the center around which human services function." Such groups as the American Association of Retired Persons, Compassionate Friends, Sudden Infant Death Syndrome groups, Geriatric Rap Program, Loving Outreach to Survivors of Suicide Victims, Stop Smoking Educational Center, New Moms, Emotional Help Anonymous, Physical Trauma groups, Family Focus, Depression Self-Help Group, Job Re-entry Therapy, Teen Challenge, and hundreds of others *in each metropolitan area alone,* are the proof.

It may even be that by the twenty-first century professional therapy for the public will be looked upon as a passing fad.

There is no doubt that a good, professional therapist can help an individual to understand and cope with certain kinds of problems much better that your neighbor next door, your mate, or your local preacher or teacher. But for *most* problems, for *most* people, there is much evidence to suggest that you'd be better off talking about it over the backyard fence and not with a shrink.

There is still another reason that informal, nonprofessional therapy has an advantage: unlike professional therapy, it does very little harm.

In most cases, it may also do very little good as well.

But this is not a putdown. *Very little* is usually *exactly* what is *needed.*

The cult of professional therapy is a straw man. What most of us need now and then is simply a little help from our friends. Yes, we must know who our friends are. And we must know how to obtain that help, and how to help them in return.

Long ago, people knew that. Long ago, there were no psychotherapists, and neither was there a violent sick world around every corner. Which is the chicken and which is the egg? Long ago, the really fine physicians would diagnose perfectly by taking a patient's history and looking at him. There were no computerized pathology labs and expert X-ray technicians. Yes, modern medical science has saved lives. And yet far fewer people feel that their lives are worth saving. They are unhappy, dependent, frustrated. To feel better physically they run to physicians whose life expectancy is several years less than the average population. To feel better mentally they run to psychotherapists whose mental health is often dubious.

But unless the buyer is very knowing, very gritty, very lucky, or all three, the buyer of mental health and emotional well-being had better beware.

26
The Secret

Many of you who read this book came to it in extreme emotional pain. Some of you will have suffered for a longer time in a possibly less piercing, but more profound, manner. As I wrote and reread *Same Time Next Week?* I pictured different people reading it, people hoping to be told what they wanted to hear, that therapy *would* usually work if only they knew this or would do that. I could feel many a reader's anguish at having that panacea taken away. But it was the purpose of *Same Time Next Week?* to replace the "answers" that never existed in the panacea that never was with real tools for making psychotherapy work, or avoiding it when it is unworkable for you.

I agree, as I have already said, that there is a handful of men and women who can make psychotherapy a glorious, irreplaceable, invaluable experience. But it is because they are *not* practicing *psychotherapy,* even though they are calling what they do by that name. They are actually participating in a relationship with another human being based upon insight, intimacy, trust, and health.

And upon *teaching.* The minority of psychotherapists who can help you do so for two reasons: (1) They are sensible, stable individuals with good intentions, who, if you sincerely want to examine your problems, may be able to do as much or more for you as anyone else would who relates to you well and honestly. (2) They *teach* you a new, productive way of looking at things.

If the therapist is seen primarily as a teacher, and not as a therapist, what he does becomes more meaningful and practical—theoretically. How often the theoretical becomes the real depends entirely on (1) whether the "therapist" explicitly (or at least implicitly) recognizes his role as teacher; (2) whether he knows what he is talking about; (3) whether there is a basic human rapport between therapist and patient—whether you "connect"; and (4) whether he can impart a knowledge of the tools of *self*-learning.

Yet no tool is better than the person who uses it.

If there is one message throughout these pages, it is that we must each fashion our own tools and our own method for using them, if we are to have ongoing emotional and mental health. This does not mean you will be free of anxiety and depression, problems and troubles. It means that, as Zorba the Greek exulted, in one sense *life* is *trouble,* and the person who truly loves life may almost hungrily confront his troubles at times. Such an attitude is anathema or heresy to most of us. Yet it is the only way, on any level of life, to leave our "same time-next week" psychic prisons.

As children we were fascinated by the radio or TV adventure tales that began with someone trying to tell the hero the secret clue. "The secret is . . .," they would say, then suddenly be shot or the hero hit on the head or whatever it took to keep the secret from being revealed secondhand.

There is incalculable wisdom in this.

For there *is* a secret. But it cannot be revealed secondhand. Because that and that alone *is* the secret.

All therapy will fail unless . . . the therapist is *you.*